MORE Than My Mountains

Endorsements

There is nothing like reading a true story with an amazing outcome. We all love to hear how the impossible situations in our life can drastically change for the good. The book you are holding in your hands is an account of the author's amazing story and survival. Reading the miracles God has performed for Whitney will bless you beyond measure. She doesn't just share her inspiring testimony; she wants you to know of others who have climbed mountains in their lives too. So, this book is also a detailed account of others who overcame tremendous tests and trials and came out victorious by the grace of God. Even though the mountains were different for each person, the result was the same. It was always worth the effort when you got to the top of the mountain and saw the view. A faith that cannot be tested is a faith that cannot be trusted. This book will unbelievably impact your life. Get ready for a blessing as people share how their personal struggles became their greatest victories through Christ, who strengthened them to climb the mountains in their life. May you read and be blessed by it.

—**Dr. Calvin Ray Evans**, pastor of Rubyville Community Church and Director of Evangelistic Outreach

Author Whitney Lane Ward has drawn from her personal journey battling a chronic illness for much of her life to create a God-inspired, inspirational message for children and others who face similar health challenges: God loves you and He hasn't abandoned you, and you are much more important to God than your illness.

—**Dr. Randal Olshefski**, section chief, Hematology and Oncology Department at Nationwide Children's Hospital, the author's specialist for twenty-two years.

I've witnessed Whitney Lane Ward from the beginning of her writing journey. With its ups and downs she has tackled every mountain. I've watched her medical journey over the last three years, and she tackles everything with the word of God and prayer.

Her book *MORE Than My Mountains* is an honest and powerful book for anyone on a difficult journey in life. If you know someone with a rare disease, difficult medical journey, or tumultuous events in their lives, this book is the book is for them.

—**Cherrilynn Bisbano**, former soldier—National Guard, author of *Shine Don't Whine*, founder of *The Write Proposal*, and co-founder of *The Write Coach*

This is the perfect combination of guidance and encouragement for readers fighting difficult battles, all while learning about the author's own inspiring story. I was diagnosed with an incurable, chronic illness at a young age, and I went through a period of feeling different than my peers and struggled to understand why I was facing such a hardship.

This book is a great tool if you are struggling with understanding why you are faced with such a huge mountain to climb, and provides the tools needed to guide you from peak to peak.

—**Heather McCutcheon**, clinical radiology facilitator and lupus warrior who cheers her daughter through her own medical conditions

When you immerse yourself in *MORE Than My Mountains*, you are able to ride the wave of feelings and emotions Whitney has experienced throughout her lifelong battle with chronic illness. No matter your struggle, Whitney's words help you relate and understand each of us have our own mountains to climb. This inspiring book will have you looking more closely at your own challenges, accepting your weaknesses, kicking them to the curb and filling your backpack (and heart) with only the necessities to help you climb higher.

—Sarah Hatfield, RN BSN CPHON

Don't we all find ourselves climbing mountains at some point in our own lives? *MORE Than My Mountains* will help you reach your own mountain peaks with grace and purpose. Author and podcaster Whitney Lane Ward has masterfully woven together the threads of her life journey with a rare, chronic disease and the threads to becoming an expert mountain climber. Through the raw, authentic way Whitney chronicles her own health challenges, we come face to face with the questions and doubts we all encounter as we scale our own mountains. Whitney brings us through healing tears of sorrow and joy, always pointing us to where our real hope is, in God. I will be sharing the invaluable riches of *MORE Than My Mountains* personally and professionally with family, friends, patients, and colleagues for years to come.

—Staci B Morgan, MSN, PNP (Pediatric Nurse Practitioner), Indiana Association of Home Educators Special Learners Team Lead, author, and fellow zebra with her own 'dazzle' (zebra herd).

Author Whitney Lane Ward uses her talent as a writer to convey how God has guided her through the highs and lows of living with chronic illness. She takes you along on her journey as she has grown, changed, and developed into the confident mountain climber God has called her to be. No matter whether you're living with chronic illness or facing other mountains of your own, her book will help you face those challenges and use them for your spiritual growth and God's ultimate glory. Whitney's raw emotions will reach out and grab you from each page, allowing you to draw parallels in your own life's experiences. Her intentions are honest, her openness is admirable, and her delivery is stellar. Whitney has given the world a gift by sharing her experiences, and there is truly something for everyone in this book. As her words draw you to explore your own valleys and mountain peaks, you will find yourself empowered, restored, and ready to climb your next mountain.

—**Misty Hawk**, nurse practitioner/primary care provider

Do you have a mountain to climb? If so, Whitney Lane Ward will show you how.

In fact, she might just climb a few steps with you. As Whitney's high school English teacher, I witnessed her struggle at the base of her mountain.

I only saw the surface of Whitney's mountain--the everyday struggle of a young woman who was extremely ill and just wanted to be normal and belong.

Read this book and let Whitney show you how to overcome. The biggest mountain is emotional—liberate your damaged self and scurry up that mountain.

—**Mary Jo Pfleger**, retired high school English teacher

Whitney Lane Ward's book will inspire you with her real-life experiences of how she has overcome challenges and has continued to put her faith in God in the midst of these mountains she has faced. After reading this book, you will understand to a greater degree that you are MORE than your mountains.

—**Joy Shearer**, elementary English language teacher

MORE Than My Mountains

Whitney Lane Ward

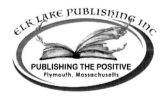

ELK LAKE PUBLISHING INC

PUBLISHING THE POSITIVE
Plymouth, Massachusetts

Scripture quotations are taken from the King James Version of the Holy Bible, in the public domain.

Cover and Interior Design: Derinda Babcock

Editor(s):Steve Mathisen, Susan K. Stewart, Deb Haggerty

Author Represented By: Cyle Young Literary Elite

PUBLISHED BY: Elk Lake Publishing, Inc., 35 Dogwood Drive, Plymouth, MA 02360, 2021s

---

Library Cataloging Data

Names: Ward, Whitney Lane (Whitney Lane Ward)

MORE Than My Mountains / Whitney Lane Ward

210 p. 23cm × 15cm (9in × 6 in.)

Identifiers: ISBN-13: 9781649494085 (paperback) | 9781649494092 (trade paperback)| 9781649494108 (e-book)

Key Words: chronic illness, autoimmune disease, disease, Christian healing, illness memoirs, overcoming challenges, emotionally healthy spirituality

Library of Congress Control Number: 2021948317 Nonfiction

DEDICATION

I dedicate this book to all my doctors and nurses. I have no doubt God ordained you all to be my caretakers during this adventure. Your wisdom and keen intuition as well as your care and dedication to me gave me the courage to climb past my limitations— even when what I attempted terrified you. I appreciate your respect for my faith and your acknowledgment of miracles. With you all and God in my corner, my disease never stood a chance.

TABLE OF CONTENTS

NOTE FROM THE AUTHOR

The mountain climbing techniques and applications the author shares are her personal interpretation of her research that she references and inspirationally applies to *life's mountains*. The information shared should not be considered an educational or expert book on climbing. If you are considering ascending a mountain, you should reach out to a climbing expert for guidance on how to begin.

FOREWORD

I can remember first learning about positive feedback loops in college biology: one initial inciting action causes a reaction. The reaction promotes more of the original, starting action. This creates a "loop" and restarts the whole process. Sometimes positive feedback loops are called virtuous cycles, or sometimes vicious cycles when the result is undesirable. The result is always a *snowball* effect, an amazing amplification of what initially was an imperceivably small event. Positive feedback loops are powerful, effective, and often self-perpetuating. They are essential for all life, allowing us to think, move, heal, and fight off infections.

During my first year of graduate school, we discovered that a genetic mutation had created a new positive feedback loop within Whitney's immune system. However, this one wasn't good. Her immune responses would begin just like they would in a normal person. One white blood cell would recognize an infection and release growth factors. The growth factors would cause that white blood cell to grow and divide. Newly formed white blood cells would release more growth factors, eventually resulting in a massive expansion of white blood cells and a robust immune response. Normally, this process would end once the infection was eradicated—however, the genetic mutation in Whitney's cells caused the cells to continue to divide even after the infection was gone. This uncontrolled immune response caused a life-threatening autoimmune disease, i.e., Whitney's immune system was attacking her own body. The discovery was an important breakthrough, which demonstrated Whitney's condition was a new disease and provided key insights that might be used to find new treatments.

While Whitney's cells were teaching the world new truths about the human immune system, Whitney's life story and response to adversity were teaching me priceless lessons about doctoring and life. Working with Whitney provided a window into the toll that a chronic disease takes on the body and mind of those affected. I'll never forget how my heart sank as I first read her medical record—a file of papers four feet tall. With each hospitalization, surgery, and test result I reviewed, I vicariously walked through her battle with an unknown disease. I felt overwhelmed and despairing as I contemplated her reality and the complete unknown of her future. In the clinic, I expected to see the embodiment of the stormy emotions I was feeling. Instead, I met a woman with a down-to-earth realism about her situation, a quiet strength, and a heart for others. I'll never forget her saying, "I hope the research helps the next person born with my disease." In one sentence, Whitney taught me a lesson that has stuck with me ever since: although we often cannot control our circumstances, our circumstances do not control us either. Or as she would put it, she is not defined by her disease. It is this truth and Whitney's example that still encourage me to do better and consider the needs of others—no matter what the circumstances.

Now, years later, Whitney continues teaching me and giving back to those around her, this time with a positive feedback loop as old as humankind. In the pages of this book, Whitney shares the story of her journey through unprecedented circumstances and how God used men and women in her life to guide her. These "mountain guides," as Whitney identifies them, not only helped her overcome her life's biggest challenges but also equipped her to guide others through their trials in life. Now Whitney pays forward the wisdom and strength her guides imparted to her in a powerful, effective, and self-perpetuating text. I hope you, too, are caught up in the snowball effect that initially empowered Whitney to overcome and now empowers her to serve as a guide to so many others.

—Dr. Ian Lamborn

ACKNOWLEDGMENTS

To My Parents:

Mom and Dad, even though I was the one fighting my disease, I know it still profoundly affected you too. When parents watch their child experience pain in their body and frightening uncertainties due to illness, it breaks their hearts in the worse possible way. They wish they could take their child's place. While your heart ached for what I endured, you always put on a brave face for my sake, encouraging me never to allow my disease to control me but to look for precious moments that would allow me to live life to the fullest. You supported my desire to surpass my limitations, even when those limitations seemed impossible to surpass. Above all, you taught me to trust God because he had a purpose for my life despite my disease. Your belief and confidence in me gave me the courage to face the unknowns surrounding me. The selfless love, dedication, and devotion you poured into me has had a profound impact on my life and helped shape me into the woman I am today. I thank God, he gave me the parents he knew I needed—the first people who showed me I am MORE!

To My Sister:

Linsay, Mom and Dad always laughed and said God knew which daughter could handle pain and medical procedures. While God gave me a high pain tolerance and the ability not to dwell on the "what if's" and unknowns, you were given the gift of compassion and a selfless heart—the sister my soul needed in the midst of heartache and confusion. Growing up, you were always there when I was sick, nursing me back to health and making sure I had what I needed. That stability in my ever-changing world was like a soothing and healing balm to my invisible wounds. You always told me I could achieve my dreams even if they seemed unobtainable to others. You were my protector and stood up to anyone who would dare to tear me down. You aren't just my sister; you're my best friend.

To My Grandma:

How I adore my silly, fun-loving, selfless Grandma! Your house was a haven for me. My life revolved around doctor's appointments and having no energy to do anything but lie on the couch, but I could come to your house to get a change of scenery that lifted my spirits. You allowed me to pour my heart out to you of the pain and weight I carried from the treatment I received from other kids—your listening ear and validation of my feelings lessened the burdens I felt and helped me keep climbing. The fact you accompanied Mom and me to almost every doctor's appointment while I was growing up meant the world to me—it took my mind off of any procedures or tests I was dreading, and I treasured the extra time I got to spend with you. Thank you for always going above and beyond to show me I matter.

To Those Who Have Gone On:

Oh, Grandpa, how I miss you! I miss our early morning garden adventures of picking corn, green beans, and tomatoes. I miss your lessons on putting out a proper garden and learning your tricks to produce a successful harvest. I miss your famous PB&J sandwiches, and your ability to fix anything. You were one of a kind, Grandpa, with a heart of gold. I will forever be grateful you accepted Jesus Christ as your Savior two weeks before you passed away, and I have the peace of knowing I will see you again!

Memaw, I can't believe it's been over sixteen years since you went home to be with Jesus. Although miles separated us, I couldn't wait every summer to visit you in Georgia, and the year you came to spend Christmas with our family in Ohio will always be a precious memory to me. I only wish we would have had more time together, but I'm so glad we will have eternity to spend together catching up!

Grandad, I was just two when you passed away, but I'm so glad you accepted Jesus as your Savior before you passed away as well because I'm so excited to get to know you!

Papaw Trim, Mamaw Marie, Papaw Alvis, and Mamaw Marg, not many people have the rare opportunity to know their great-grandparents, but I did. Thank you for the rich heritage you left in my life!

Special thanks to all my friends and family who allowed me to share their stories and how they impacted my life. I would also like to thank my agent, Del Duduit, who has walked me through the publishing process, answering all of my questions, and calming all of my worry.

Lastly, I'd like to send my profound appreciation to Deb Haggerty, for believing in me and making my dream of becoming a published author come true, and to my editors, Susan and Steve, and my graphic designer, Derinda Babcock—thank you for working hard to make my book all I hoped it would be.

INTRODUCTION

I sat in Asbury University's student center chatting with my friend Kelli. She was just about to finish her shift working the desk, and we had plans to have dinner together in the cafeteria. A girl we both knew walked up to us.

"Hey, Kelli and Whitney."

"Hello," we said in return.

We talked about random subjects, catching up on the buzz of the campus, when suddenly, the girl grabbed my hand that had a patch of psoriasis on top of it. "That looks just like the scar the guy had on *Fight Club!*" she said in excitement.

I wasn't excited. I was mortified. The last person I wanted to be compared to was a sweaty, grungy, beaten-up man who fought in an underground club. My heart felt chafed and raw like a scrape when the air hits the sore.

I laughed awkwardly, and Kelli's eyes were wide—shocked the girl would have the boldness to say something so hurtful. My friend changed the subject, and even though the girl's comments stung, I felt relieved no one else was around to hear her belittle my deformities that made me feel vulnerable and insecure.

During our conversation, two guys walked up and asked Kelli for equipment for some of the recreational activities available in the student center. As Kelli searched for the items they requested, the girl struck up a conversation with the two guys she apparently knew, but I had no idea who they were. Kelli returned and gave them what they needed and then gathered her stuff for us to leave to head over to the cafeteria. I started to get up from my seat.

"Hey!" I fell forward with the unexpected force as the girl grabbed my wrist once again without my permission. "Doesn't this scar on her hand look like the one from *Fight Club?*" She pulled my hand close to the guys for their inspection.

"Oh, yeah!" one said.

Tears began to bubble in the corners of my eyes. I felt so ugly and undesirable. Kelli had had enough. Before they could fawn and analyze my psoriasis any more, Kelli grabbed my arm. "We are leaving!" she said forcibly, telling them the conversation was over with the coldness of her tone. As we walked away, Kelli put her arm around me, "You are amazing," she whispered. I appreciated her words, but I didn't feel amazing at that moment. I felt like a freak of nature people saw as "less than"—some*thing* to be pitied.

When I got back to my room after dinner, I allowed the tears I had bottled up for the last hour to stream down my face. I had made such progress of claiming and believing my worth, but in one moment, the feelings I had growing up of insecurity, doubt, pain, not being enough, and the daggers of people's hurtful words came flooding into my soul like a strong current that bursts through a dam.

As the tears continued to flow in my dark dorm room, my eyes rested on my Bible. *I need something, Lord,* I pleaded. I opened my Bible and allowed the pages to randomly fall. My eyes connected with John 1:3— "All things were made by him; and without him was not any thing made that was made." My tears turned from tears of heartbreak to tears of peace. God gently whispered to my battered soul—*Rest assured, I made you, and I see the beautiful woman you are. Rest assured you are my treasured creation, and you are MORE than enough.*

Ironically, way before I learned my disease was caused by a rare gene mutation and had the honor of naming it a Latin word that meant "more," God's message to me over and over was you are MORE. It took me years to heal from the pain caused by others and my disease, but the strength and assurance I was MORE than my mountains always resonated deep within my soul, giving me the perseverance to keep climbing because of who God created me to be.

That's why I felt called to share my story with you. Through my journey of overcoming disease and the stories of my fellow mountain climbers ascending toward mountain-top victories, my hope and prayers are you'll see yourself how God sees you. Despite the mountains looming over you of anxiety, fear, and self-doubt crushing you like an iron fist, God sees the beautiful confidence, faith, and assurance within you, ready to bloom like a vast field of flowers encompassing your mountain-top views. I invite you to join me on this climb to healing and a newfound understanding of God's miraculous grace and who he created you to be—MORE than your mountains.

THE MOUNTAIN PEAK

When your strength comes from the right source, there's not a mountain you can't climb. —Whitney Lane Ward

September 9, 2016—I felt my heartbeat through my dress as I sat in the lecture hall at the University of Pennsylvania. I'd awaited this day since my journey began five years ago at the National Institutes of Health (NIH) in Bethesda, Maryland.

To a small-town girl, the university classroom seemed large and imposing as I sensed the air of greatness it held. I watched as men and women filed in buzzing with excitement about the upcoming presentation on the breakthroughs in medical research.

Ian Lamborn was ready to defend his dissertation—the speech everyone came to watch and celebrate. I held a silent role no one else could claim. I was the subject of Ian's dissertation.

Am I a nonprofit CEO? A wonderful humanitarian? A specialist of the illiterate, who helps children unlock the wonderful world of words? I am none of these. My accomplishment illuminates the fact a higher power exists.

I was the only known person alive with the rare gene mutation and the reason for Ian's immunological dissertation.

As I sat with my parents and sister, I listened to Ian discuss my medical journey, which included abnormal

B-cells, T-cells, and how my body's messaging system didn't communicate properly. He shared with the room of doctors and medical students about the hemolytic crises and the deformities for any patient with this disease.

As he spoke, each symptom and medical phenomenon reminded me of the stolen parts of my life—yet joy filled my soul. I was alive and well enough to attend Ian's dissertation. What a miracle.

These good and perfect gifts were from the Father above. God gave me the strength to fight. He empowered me with the perseverance and drive to keep climbing despite what seemed to be insurmountable odds.

At the end of Ian's dissertation, he thanked everyone who assisted him in the research process and explained he had one particular person he wanted to thank. Me! He looked at me as he explained the voluminous amount of blood drawn. He spoke about the bizarre tests I endured, such as the blister study test where a mechanism was placed on my forearm that suctioned my skin for an hour and formed eight tiny blisters. The liquid of each blister was drained, the surface of the blisters removed, and then the blister liquid was placed into the sores on my arm. This test caused my hand to swell to three times its size. The results of the process showed Ian the low degree to which my white blood cells fight off infection.

"You know we choose our dissertation subjects based on how easy they and their families are to work with. We choose them because of their willingness to put themselves through tests and research. She fit both criteria. This woman went above and beyond and did everything I asked of her, even when she knew she wasn't obligated to do so," he said with a smile. "She totally understood all of the tubes of blood she gave, and the weird research tests she put herself through wouldn't only help her, but others diagnosed with this rare gene mutation. She is a huge part of why I am here today."

After he spoke, he picked up a bouquet from behind the lectern, walked over, and gave the flowers to me along with a hug. A realization swept over me. I gained something I didn't know I needed—something I realized I didn't have until this moment—closure.

Everything I endured was worth it. My heart bloomed with the profound revelation of what God created me to be, MORE. MORE than my disease, MORE than my pain, MORE than my mountains.

In my mind, as the sunlight glistened on the mountaintop that had seemed unreachable, I gazed at the valleys below. I smiled because there was a time I didn't know if I would make it to the first plateau. My disease made it seem like the dark valley would remain a constant for me, and I wouldn't be able to climb out and experience my life. What I saw from the mountaintop applauded me from the valley below—my beginning. The cheers of accomplishment echoed through the valley—*you are MORE!*

The most challenging aspect of climbing a mountain is gaining the courage to begin the journey. The insecurities and doubts swarmed my thoughts before I even started my ascent with writing these words you are reading now. As with each draft I wrote of this book, I struggled to know where to start each chapter and questioned what I should share. I was responsible for piecing together the different peaks of my mountains to encourage you no matter how the mountain you face weighed on me. My deepest desire was not to merely share inspirational, feel-good stories but also to share the mountain climbing tools I'd found essential as I embarked on this tumultuous journey. My desire is for you to walk away from my words knowing you are MORE and knowing the God who gives strength to reach the pinnacle.

When mountains loom before me, how do I begin the climb? How do I rise and make it to the top? What if the mountains are difficult classes with jagged rocks and uneven terrain causing me to stumble? No matter the type of mountain I face, whether it comes from my chronic illness or being brave enough to reveal my vulnerability on paper, one tangible fact of life remains constant. The key to start is to put one foot in front of the other. It doesn't matter the height of the mountain. If your strength comes from the right source, there's not a mountain you can't climb with God as your power.

My question is—will you tap into God's power source? Will you begin the trek from the valley of fear and insecurity to the elevations of self-realization and growth? God's power is never ending and uniquely special. He created you for a purpose. Also, I am here to help you. Even when the atmosphere starts to thin as we near the highest altitude and victory is so close, I will be here to guide you and cheer for you. We'll gaze at the spectacular mountain views and then look down at the sharp cliffs you overcame, and you'll see what I saw—your beginning applauding you and saying—You Are MORE.

MOUNTAIN GUIDE TO THE NEXT PEAK:

1. Describe the mountain before you.
2. What holds you back from beginning the climb?
3. Why do you think those doubts, fears, and insecurities cripple you?
4. Think about tapping into God's strength. What would you ask him?
5. Envision the summit—the highest point of the mountain. What is your beginning and why will it applaud you?

_____

_____

_____

_____

_____

_____

_____

_____

_____

_____

_____

_____

_____

_____

_____

_____

_____

_____

_____

LIFELINE TO THE TOP

Come unto me, all ye that labour and are heavy laden, and I will give you rest. Take my yoke upon you, and learn of me; for I am meek and lowly in heart: and ye shall find rest unto your souls. For my yoke is easy, and my burden is light. —Jesus of Nazareth (Matthew 11:28-30)

Hands were raised to volunteer, and I wanted to be included.

My sister, Linsay, didn't raise her hand so I could do this on my own. At the age of five, I loved being my big sister's shadow, but at times, her overprotective nature made me feel the need for independence.

"Oh, Whitney, you have your hand raised, so you come with us too," said my children's church teacher.

Oh yay! They picked me, and we get to leave the room.

I followed the other kids to the room next door and sat. To my disappointment, we weren't chosen to be special helpers. Instead, the teacher taught another lesson. I didn't understand what was going on and I needed to go to the bathroom.

"Yes, Whitney, do you have a question?" The teacher looked at my little hand in the air.

"Can I go to the bathroom?"

The woman sighed. "Are you sure you can't hold it, sweetie?"

I shook my head and crossed and uncrossed my legs to show the urgency. Even at my young age, I was aware adults didn't always believe me when I said I had to go to the bathroom. I went often, so they thought I used a full bladder as an excuse to get up and roam around. My validation came a year later when doctors told me my enlarged spleen pressed against my bladder and caused the frequent urges to go.

I walked back from the bathroom to the sanctuary. The service was over, and I wanted to find my family. My mom walked toward me with tears in her eyes and her face glowing with joy.

She wrapped her arms around me. "Whitney, Linsay told me you got saved. I'm so proud of you, honey."

My little brain didn't know what she was talking about, but I knew this—my teacher took the students into the other room to get saved, and I couldn't bear to tell my mom I left in the middle of the teacher's invitation. I smiled, but my heart knew I'd missed out on something special.

Two years later, Miss Carole asked if anyone wanted to come and pray. I remembered how two girls a little bit older than me asked Jesus to come into their hearts. Miss Carole had them stand up front, she put her arm around them, and she announced the decision they made to all the children in the room. The beam on her face, the applauding, and the congratulations from friends were what I wanted to experience. So I went to the altar and uttered a few words in prayer, but my biggest hope was people would be happy and pleased with what I did. After I prayed, I was celebrated, my friends and teachers applauded me, but again, something was missing.

When a child endures chronic illness, the insecurities, self-doubt, and internal scars take root in their hearts, even if they are not aware. The effects cause them to miss out, and they often feel left out. I couldn't voice the feeling as a child, but I desperately desired not to be left out but to be let in.

Three years later, I finally heard the unseen calling at my church's spring revival, the sweet invitation from Jesus Christ, my Savior. I finally understood I had never been left out. God was always right there to let me in. I didn't want to go to a big altar and be surrounded by a bunch of adults, so I drew from past experiences—I went to the bathroom. In the stall, I asked Jesus to come into my heart and to forgive my sins. No applauding, no words of congratulations, just me, and a sweet assurance from God that I'm accepted by him.

Mountain climbers through the ages have experienced harrowing escapades. One of the most famous mountain climbs in history comes to mind—Abraham and Isaac's trek up Mount Moriah. After years of waiting, God had gifted Abraham with a son. Then God commanded Abraham to take Isaac to the top of Mount Moriah and offer him as a sacrifice. I'm not a Christian who claims to understand everything in the Bible, but in my heart and mind, I couldn't fathom why God, who condemned murder and child sacrifice as barbaric and evil, had instructed Abraham to sacrifice his son. It seemed contradictory.

I imagined the scene. All boy, Isaac runs ahead, throws rocks, and chatters without taking a breath about the peculiar birds he saw perched on the trees and what adventure awaits him. He sees this mountain climb as a grand quest with his father. Yet, Abraham's steps feel weighted. It is a struggle for him to put one foot in front of the other. His father's smiles encourage Isaac's exuberance, but on the inside, a storm rages. Abraham had a choice to make as he climbed this mountain. Did he preserve the life of the son he loved more than anything? Or did he obey the God who gave him everything?

God never intended for Abraham to end his son's life. God wanted Abraham to trust in him and gave him the strength to climb the mountain. My God isn't cruel—he operates in grace and mercy. You see, God knew what was on top of the mountain waiting for Abraham—his lifeline.

What a beautiful sight it must have been, as Abraham shouted with joy and relief when he heard the bleating of the ram! God provided another sacrifice for Abraham.

I don't have to wonder if I have a lifeline. When God sent his son Jesus Christ to die on the cross for all of humanity's sins, he became the lifeline for all of us. John the Baptist said it so profoundly when he first saw Jesus, "Behold, the Lamb of God who takes away the sin of the world." (John 1:29)

When I asked Jesus to be my Savior when I was ten, I tapped into the sustaining strength of my heavenly Father. Did I get better after I made this decision? No, the opposite—I got sicker. But I claimed faith over fear, determined to choose better instead of bitter. His joy in me helped me focus on what I could do instead of the pain and what I couldn't do.

My disease never defined me. Instead, I defined my illness when I surpassed the foretold limitations. I didn't just want to exist—I wanted to live. Sure, the footholds, valleys, and cliffs I will share with you gave me scrapes, bruises, and cuts, but I could climb because of my strong and enduring lifeline.

Who is your lifeline? How do you make it to the top of your mountains? I can't decide this for you, but I can tell you when I accepted Christ's free gift of eternal life, it was the best decision I ever made. All I did was ask him to come into my heart and forgive me for the wrong I had done in my life, and I received a never-ending supply of God's strength.

If you feel a drawing whisper in the depths of your soul, my prayer is you will accept it, so when you stand at the bottom of your mountains wondering how you'll be able to climb, you'll hear the distant calling of your lifeline at the top telling you, "come to me, and I will help you."

MOUNTAIN GUIDE TO THE NEXT PEAK:

1. Do you remember when God saved you? How has God's strength helped you climb your mountains?
2. List some of the scrapes, bruises, and scars caused by the cliffs you've climbed. It may be painful to remember, but you will stand in awe, recalling what you endured so you could receive what you have now.
3. How did your strong and enduring lifeline give you the strength you needed to keep climbing despite the scrapes, bruises, and scars?

_____

_____

_____

_____

_____

_____

_____

_____

_____

_____

_____

_____

_____

_____

_____

_____

_____

_____

BORN TO CLIMB

The summit is what drives us, but the climb itself is
what matters. —Conrad Anker

It was a long black velvet dress.

The buttons were in an even row and the focal point of
the gown. The golden trim around my wrists added a simple
and sophisticated look. In my seven-year-old mind, I felt
so grown-up. It was the perfect dress, and when the day
came, I wanted to be buried in it.

I was aware of my mortality on a conscience level. My
situation was black and white in my eyes, as it is with most
children.

I struggled between handling adult issues and looking
at the mountain before me with resilient innocence. I
accepted the fact I could die soon. The dress I loved filled
me with a safe and secure self-assurance that gave me the
feeling of a reprieve from the finality. The scary unknowns
and uncertain future never immobilized me with fear. They
did the opposite.

I was a spunky, quick-witted, sassy, and stubborn
little girl. My childhood nickname was "Punky Brewster"
(named after a character in an 80's sitcom of the same
name). I embraced my style and individuality no matter
what others thought. This confidence gave my young soul

the determination to live life to the fullest—even if my story ended at "once upon a time."

The tenacity and courage God had knitted into me burst forth—I wasn't born to succumb to the mountain—I was born to climb it. Even if my grim and frail beginning told me otherwise.

One Friday afternoon, this free spirit ran in the vast green pastures and climbed haylofts at my great-grandpa's farm, not realizing the next morning, my life would change forever.

Brilliant blue skies contrasted with the red-hot pain I felt within me. Every movement caused fiery darts of agony to shoot through my legs, connecting to a perfect bullseye in my kneecap. "I can't move my legs."

Just as we look back and see prophetic words that foreshadowed traumatic events, those five words, "I can't move my legs," were the sounds of my Shofar, just as it was blown in Biblical times when it was time to fight a war. My battle had begun.

The next two days were a whirlwind of doctors' appointments and tests. I entered a scary world I hadn't known existed. My parents shuffled me from my local emergency room to Cincinnati Children's Orthopedic Department and then to Cincinnati Children's Rheumatology Clinic. I felt like we'd fallen into a deep rabbit hole with no return.

As I sat on the examination table, I saw vibrant colors splashed the walls. Even as a six-year-old, I handled everything with a quiet, level-headed strength, even though the fears and questions swirled like a tornado within the depths of my soul.

The door creaked open and broke the silence. A tall man with black hair walked in. Behind him was a woman who radiated warmth. His kind eyes met mine, and then he looked at my parents.

"You know I wasn't supposed to be here today. I was supposed to be at a rheumatology conference."

Tears filled my mother's eyes. "Oh yes, you are supposed to be here. A higher power ordained this."

The man lowered his head then focused his attention on me. He extended his hand, and I shook it, instantly responding to his friendly demeanor.

"Hello, I'm Dr. M. You're Whitney Ward, aren't you?"

I hunched my shoulders and nodded with a grin. My new doctor smiled—instantly melting to my reaction. As a tinier than usual six-year-old, people often saw me as a live baby doll they wanted to cuddle.

"Well, in that case, I think I'm going to call you WW Square."

For the first time since I uttered those five words, warm feelings wrapped their arms around me with a hug of security. Two truths took root in my young heart. First, Dr. M wouldn't just be my doctor, he would be my friend, and second, because of his friendship, the mountain didn't seem as monstrous. Now, I could climb.

My assistant pastor once taught a lesson on how to climb a mountain. I was so intrigued by what he shared, I asked him where he found his information. He directed me to an article he found on *wikiHow*, entitled "How to Climb a Mountain." According to the website, one of the most important initiatives someone can do before they climb is to find a good guide. This is essential if a climber is attempting to ascend a mountain not within their climbing skill set.[1]

"If I were to go to the New River Gorge, West Virginia, or Horseshoe Canyon in Arkansas, I would not get a guide but only buy a guidebook, because I would only be doing sport climbing and the rock is similar to here. I would definitely get a guide if I were planning something outside of my skill level, such as multi-pitch, mountaineering, or Trad. I would also get a guide if I were on a strange or off the beaten path area." Greg Botzet, who has been sport climbing for nine years, explained.

wikiHow also encourages potential climbers to join climbing clubs and classes to gain invaluable information to assist with honing the skills for the type of mountain they are climbing. The benefits of joining a mountain climbing club are networking with other climbers, and gleaning wisdom from their mountain experiences. Clubs will even organize group climbs for beginners to intermediate climbers. Hands-on experiences and interactions such as this provide learning and knowledge you can't always get from a book.[1]

The same application applies to the mountains not in our skill set or off the beaten path. We must have an excellent guide who will ignite the fire of courage within us. Having someone who understands what it takes to climb the specific mountain we are facing is crucial.

God has placed many guides to help me climb my mountains, but Dr. M holds a special place in my heart because he was the first guide on my uphill medical journey, and he gave me my beloved nickname the day my life became a revolving door of frightening unknowns. Then, he gave me good news. A drug, Naprosyn, treated septic arthritis.

"If all patients responded this well to this drug as Whitney has, rheumatologists would be out of a job," my rheumatologist said for comedic relief.

During this time, I met doctors whose specialties I didn't know existed and could certainly not pronounce. Unfortunately, my rheumatologist also delivered the bad news.

"All the tests came back negative, WW Square," Dr. M said.

We didn't know why my white blood count quadrupled or why my body was anemic with low hemoglobin. Doctors were at a loss as to why my spleen was the largest spleen most doctors ever experienced. It was a mystery why my immune system couldn't fend off infections or calm the raging diseases within.

My parents could celebrate—I didn't have cancer, MS, lupus, or CF. However, without a diagnosis, Dr. M could not create a successful treatment plan. Any treatment explored was a roller coaster of trial and error, not a permanent solution. Regardless, my parents remained strong for me and cheered me through another needle stick, CT scan, or MRI while processing what a life-threatening undiagnosed disease could mean for their little girl.

My parents did their best to stay as light-hearted as possible. They enticed me to giggle and smile any chance they got while I laid in the hospital bed as the unknowns swirled around me. I remember one day, my dad put his dry sense of humor to use.

Knock, knock, knock-another white coat at my hospital room door.

"Excuse me, Mr. and Mrs. Ward? I'm one of the residents. I was wondering if I could feel Whitney's spleen. My colleagues tell me I'll never feel another spleen as large as hers again." The nervousness and humbleness in the young doctor's stance were proof he was still a small fish in a big pond, not yet able to gauge reactions from his patient's parents.

My father picked up on this and initiated a little fun.

"Yeah, we don't care, but a lot of you have been in and out of Whitney's room just to feel her spleen, and sometimes there's even been a line of doctors outside in the hall just waiting for their turn. So, my wife and I decided we could make a little money from this, and we're going to start charging every doctor a quarter who wants to feel our daughter's spleen."

The doctor's face became as white as the sheets wrapped around my small frame. "Well, I don't think I, well that is sir, I don't think I'm allow—"

My mother took pity on the poor soul. "Oh, dear, I'm sorry. My husband likes to joke. Go ahead, honey. If Whitney is okay with it, you can examine her."

Dad and I laughed as Mom's look told us we would get a tongue lashing after the doctor left. "Yeah, I'm sorry. But, with these circumstances, you have to find ways to laugh," Dad made peace with the doctor.

Our little family clung to every glimpse of joy and light moments. The hospitals and doctor visits were a new normal. We needed to navigate the climb, and Dr. M became our guide.

He had a white, dry erase board covered in hypotheses of what could be wreaking havoc on my body. In addition, the doctor held countless round table discussions with his colleagues, brainstorming different diseases with similar attributes.

The most remarkable characteristic he exemplified as a guide was his care for me. My mother and I made many trips to doctor's appointments after the discovery of my undiagnosed disease. But I never felt I was going to a doctor's appointment. I was going to see my friends. Dr. M always walked into my room, looked at my mom, and said these words, "Okay, Mom, you stay seated and don't make a peep. WW Square and I need to have a conversation first." And we did. He asked me about my big sister, how school was going, and if I'd bought any new shoes.

God loves me so much he gave me strength and a kind and compassionate guide who used all his medical expertise and resources to keep me alive. With this team, I had the courage to face the peaks and footholds awaiting me. I knew I was born to climb.

What I love about God is he will give anyone the perfect guide to provide what they, his children, need and the strength to start the steep mountainside.

In June of 2019, at a writing conference, God whispered an idea into my heart—begin a show called *Mountain Climbers*. I wanted to provide a safe place where people could share their stories in a real and raw way. As I've listened to the men and women, I found many had a mountain guide.

This realization couldn't be any truer for Tom and Mindy Martin, who were my guests on *Mountain Climbers* in August 2019. Tom and Mindy took a cavern of caves once used for drugs and witchcraft and turned them into a ministry that changed countless lives in Scioto County, Ohio (nearly 100 miles east of Cincinnati). In the fall, they put on a production called *Cavern of Choices*. The drama depicts teens making choices which either bear fruit or consequences. Hundreds of people give their lives to Christ every year. During the Christmas season, they turn the cave into a winter wonderland, depicting the glory and awe of the birth of Christ. The beauty and majesty of the scenes have gained national recognition, and people from all over the country come to our small town to see it. For Easter 2021, they debuted the "Easter Cave," showing the miraculous story of Christ's crucifixion and resurrection.

They seemed like the perfect power couple—like nothing could stop them from sharing the gospel.

And yet, divorce almost did.

Tom, driven by power, money, and prestige, would often put his family last. One day, God spoke to Mindy and told her to leave.

"I heard God say, very clearly, 'You leave, and I'll work on him while you're gone'," Mindy shared. She knew an empty house would speak louder to her husband than words.

Mindy left Tom a note and took their two small children to her mom's house. Tom came home from work, saw the message, and called Mindy, thinking she and the kids were visiting Mindy's mother. But, instead, Tom received the blow of his life when he called his wife, and she revealed to him she was separating from him.

Tom chuckled and lowered his head in sad remembrance. "When she told me why she'd left, I just knew. I just knew the jig was up, and it confirmed to me the emptiness I had been feeling. One of the greatest gifts the Lord gives men and women is their children. I mean, I loved Mindy, but your kids will get you past yourself. I knew they were worth changing for—fighting for."

Tom and Mindy needed a guide, and God gave them one. Two weeks after Mindy left Tom, God led her to a Christian marriage counselor in Minnesota who was willing to spend a week with them. That week was the most exhausting and emotional week of the couple's life. The counselor guided Tom and Mindy past thick solid walls of pain, insecurities, and pride. Still, that time was the turning point and gave Tom and Mindy the courage they needed to climb their mountain. God used the guide to help save Tom and Mindy's marriage.

It's people like my beloved doctor and this marriage counselor who have the biggest impact on people and push them not to quit so those people can impact others. Now, God can use them as mountain guides.

Here's something I've discovered about the start of mountain climbing. At some point, the thrill and celebration fade, and the cliffs close in around you. When you're genuinely committed to making it to the top of your mountain, you often must lose to gain.

MOUNTAIN GUIDE TO THE NEXT PEAK:

1. Who has been a mountain guide in your life? How were they instrumental in giving you the courage to climb your mountain?
2. If it hadn't been for the guide God placed in your life, do you think you would give up? Would you have ever faced your mountain?
3. How can you be a mountain guide to others?

_____

_____

_____

_____

_____

_____

_____

_____

_____

_____

_____

_____

_____

_____

_____

_____

_____

_____

CLIMBING RESTRICTIONS

When you feel like quitting, remember why you started.
—John Di Lemme

"Please, Grandma, let me do it myself just one time!"

"But honey, I don't want you to hurt yourself. You can sit with your friends but let me run for you."

I looked at the rest of my kindergarten class sitting in a circle, ready for a game of *duck, duck, goose,* after a long day of being quiet on a field trip. We were ready to let loose. Not that I had much energy to spare.

My grandma, one of the chaperones, watched me. She didn't want the long day to do anything to cause my already fragile body to fail. But what my grandma didn't realize was I desired to grasp every milestone, every sense of normalcy, as tightly as I could because the events that created those precious memories were slipping away.

"I can do it, Grandma. Please, I'll be okay." My big blue eyes pleaded with her.

Grandma sighed. "Okay, but just one time."

I ran to my open spot with anticipation and sat. My heartbeat as the girl tapped heads, sure I would be the goose.

Duck ... Duck ... *Goose*!

I jumped up and ran. I had something to prove. I relished the wind in my hair and the sun shining on my face in approval. I plopped in my spot just before the other girl could beat me there. I smiled at my grandma in triumphant victory. I did it. I fought for this moment, and I flew like an eagle.

In my formative years, it seemed like I experienced one loss after another. I knew I was born to climb the mountain, but as a little girl, I faced the cliffs, rocks, and inclines that restricted my path to mountaintop views. Yes, I basked exultantly in every limitation I surpassed, overjoyed by the rare opportunity to live like a healthy child and play a light-hearted game of duck, duck, goose. It was a highlight in my young life because I loved being active—something which didn't pair well with a weak immune system.

My mom often says if I hadn't developed my disease, I would have been her athlete. I was fast, quick, and sturdy. My five-year-old T-ball career was proof. Lead, follow, or get out of the way was my motto. I stood at my base, ready to blaze a trail around the bases to home plate when the next batter hit the ball off the tee. *Smack!* I took off, ready to hit the home plate and high-five my coach. I faced one problem. The boy in front of me was not running fast enough and blocked me from my victory. At five, my thought process was *go faster, go faster, go faster! If he won't go faster, I'll go faster right past him.* And I did. I ran past him with all my might, determined nothing would keep me from my goal. My feet landed on home base, and I flew into my coach's arms, exclaiming, "I beat him, I beat him!" I still chuckle watching the home video of that time. The hilarity of the little boy's wide eyes and the double-take he did when he realized I had passed him was pure gold.

I loved T-ball. It gave me an adrenaline high, but my elation came crashing down the night my parents gave me some heartbreaking news.

"Whitney, sweetie, I'm so sorry, but Mommy and Daddy can't let you play T-ball anymore," my mom shared with watery eyes.

"But why?" I couldn't understand or fathom not playing the first sport I loved.

"You know how there's a lot of dirt on the field?" Dad asked.

With wide and solemn eyes, I nodded my head.

"Well, when you and your teammates run, it stirs the dirt up, and you breathe it. That dirt is making your asthma worse, honey. Your doctor says you can't be around the dirt anymore."

I didn't scream, cry, or throw a tantrum. Instead, I processed this first climbing restriction with sad acceptance, unaware many more awaited me. Quitting T-ball hurt my heart, but I don't think I comprehended there would be much more I would have to give up.

My asthma wasn't my only Achilles' heel. So was my enlarged spleen. The enormity of the diseased organ wreaked havoc on my life. Because of its size, my rib cage did not protect it, and there was a constant threat it could rupture. My rheumatologist warned a ruptured spleen could be deadly. Learning to ride a bike without training wheels became forbidden. In my attempt to master a two-wheeler, I could lose my balance, and the handlebars could swing into my left side. Organized sports became a huge no-no because a ball could slam into my left side, or another player could accidentally elbow me.

My sweet parents saw these obstacles and did everything they could to give me a normal childhood full of memories while being safe and respecting my doctors' wishes.

Every so often, my dad, sister, and I played catch in our front yard. Whenever the neighborhood kids ran into our yard asking if they could play with us, dad told them no, but they could watch if they wanted.

One day, my dad let my sister and I take turns batting.

"All right, girls, this is the last one. Whitney just went, so Linsay, you're up."

"Aw, c'mon, Dad, just a little bit longer!" Our big blue and green eyes pleaded. We knew we had our dad wrapped around our little fingers, but today Dad's tender heart toward his girls had a stronger will.

"No, we've been out long enough. It's time to go in." As much as I loved playing hard, my dad knew too much exertion could make my immune system crash, so he limited my activity.

Linsay grabbed the bat, and my dad threw the ball. She swung back, ready to connect with the ball and splat! The bat connected with me on my vulnerable left side.

I doubled over—the impact took my breath. My overprotective sister burst into tears, horrified at what she'd just done, and my dad ran to me, scooped me up, and took me into the house. My parents laid me on the bed and looked at the side where my angry organ resided. The swollen redness indicated my enormous spleen was irritated. My parents were rattled. This was the first time anything like this had happened. My mother called Cincinnati Children's and spoke to the on-call specialist. They advised my parents to take me to the local ER for a CAT scan to assess the situation. A plan needed to be put into place before I traveled two and a half hours to the Cincinnati ER.

The local ER doctor examined me.

"Okay, I have all the information I need, but with Whitney's complicated case, I want to confer with her specialist at Cincinnati Children's and make sure he agrees with my treatment plan. Mom, who do I need to call?"

"Her rheumatologist, Dr. M at Cincinnati Children's."

The doctor wrote the information, snapped his pen, and gathered his notes. "Okay, I will call him and be back shortly."

We waited, and Mom and Dad occasionally asked me how I felt.

Knock, Knock—the doctor poked their head in my room. "I have Whitney's doctor on the phone, and we both agree a CAT scan needs to be done for us to get a better picture of how the organ looks. We'll get that ordered. Mrs. Ward, could you come with me? Whitney's doctor wants to speak with you."

My mom followed, knowing and dreading what was to come. She later shared the conversation with me.

"Hello?"

"What are you doing down there!?" Dr. M bellowed.

"I know. I'm so sorry. We were so careful. Whitney's dad and sister were playing with her. We never let anyone else play with Whitney. Brent and I want to give her those chances to make memories."

The CAT scan showed my spleen didn't rupture, and I would be fine. My family and I were so relieved, but we learned a profound lesson.

As I grew, my parents could set the most secure parameters to keep me safe, but it wouldn't keep my mountain climb from being treacherous. Sometimes the limitations I tried to conquer would come with a cost, but unsurpassed limitations never enabled me to stop climbing.

Annie Wilslowski wrote an excellent article for *Climbing* magazine in 2017. The PhD nurse and climber studies high altitude illnesses. She explains that when a climber reaches a high altitude, they may experience altitude sickness. High altitude begins at 4,921 feet. The higher a person climbs, the thinner the air becomes. This causes the body to take in less oxygen. There are three levels of altitude sickness—acute mountain sickness, high-altitude pulmonary edema, with high-altitude cerebral edema being the worst. Altitude sickness is the most common climbing restriction, happening to beginners and seasoned climbers alike. Symptoms range from nausea, fatigue, headache, dizziness, cough, shortness of breath, increased heart rate, and frightening signs like confusion and personality changes with high-altitude cerebral edema.[1]

The more I inched up my mountain, the thinner the air became, and I battled the "dizziness, nausea, and fatigue."

The restrictions made me sick, but I still tried to climb higher.

My cousins, sister, and I couldn't get enough of each other, and it didn't take long once we were together for a wrestling match to ensue on my grandma's living room floor. And every time, our play was cut short when one of my cousin's knees or elbows got too close to my spleen.

Amidst our giggles and shrieks, my aunt's frantic voice rang. "Watch her spleen, watch her spleen! You know what? It's time to quit and play something else."

We all groaned in protest. "Aunt Cheryl, please, we can keep playing. I promise I'm fine. I won't get hurt."

My aunt smiled and patted my arm. "I'm sorry, sweetie, we just can't take a chance."

But I climbed until I reached the next restriction—school attendance. My fragile immune system couldn't handle a full day, and most days, I would go late. By second grade, I missed anywhere from seventy-five to one hundred days of school a year, and my little eight-year-old heart broke.

One day in the second grade, we were getting ready for parents' night. My classmates and I chattered, and our scurrying testified to our excitement to show our parents what we were learning and all our unique art. That night, my dad accompanied me while my mom joined my sister with her extracurricular activities.

I led my dad to my classroom, excited to show him my accomplishments. I saw the wall lacked my special art piece because the projects displayed were created after I left school for the day. It stung not to see my artwork on the wall with my classmates, but the pain subsided because I was distracted by the fact there were cookies in the cafeteria. My dad stayed behind to talk to my teacher while I went to the cafeteria to satisfy my sweet tooth. The cookies were gone. I gasped for breath. I felt so alone and left out—no artwork on the wall to admire and no cookies to enjoy. I ran to my classroom and flung myself into my dad's arms, sobbing on his shoulder. My teacher and father tried to calm me.

"Whitney, what's wrong?" My dad pleaded with me to tell him what made me so upset.

"Maybe someone said something to her?" My teacher wondered.

My sobs shook my body, my heart too wounded to speak. They couldn't understand why I shed tears, and I didn't know how to tell them not getting a cookie triggered an onslaught of emotions over what I had lost.

My *Mountain Climbers* guests—dear friend Danielle Hannah and her husband, Casey, are familiar with the effects of altitude sickness. They determined they would raise their kids to serve the Lord, and he blessed Casey and Danielle's desire.

"The first time we tried, I got pregnant. Everything was easy for us. The pregnancy was easy. Everything was good." Danielle shared.

A few years later, Casey and Danielle wanted another child. Since the first pregnancy went smoothly, they thought they could expect the same. But, after an ectopic pregnancy and two miscarriages, the couple wondered if they would have any more children. "It was hard. I really tried to focus on the fact I have one healthy child." Danielle said, remembering her pain.

Whether caused by physical mountains or one of life's mountains, altitude sickness is difficult to face. But how is it combated? By pre-acclimatization, Annie Wilslowski explains. This means for one to eight weeks before a climber tackles a mountain, they mimic higher altitudes with the environment they have around them by hiking and elevated sleeping.[1] Staying hydrated is also important to combating altitude sickness. The HydraPak Company (a company that designs and produces hydration systems) shares in their blog that high elevations cause the body to work harder. A climber's respiration increases, urination becomes more frequent, and the thirst response stops, thus increasing the possibility of dehydration. In fact, the body loses water faster in this environment than it would at sea level, often leading to dehydration. A climber must replace bodily fluids with water and electrolytes.[2]

Avid hiker Ryan McClay shared his experience, "I can tell you when you are acclimating, lots of water twenty-four hours beforehand is probably as critical as anything to avoid altitude sickness." In addition, this strategy helps the climber's body be introduced to higher altitudes, so when it's time for their trip, their body is more prepared for what the mountain holds.

How can we apply this strategy to the mountains we face in life? By focusing on the joy and not the pain. By choosing *can* over *cannot*. If we look at what we've lost, we'll never keep climbing. With each trial, the harder I fought to climb, the more I gained.

So, I savored the moments I played ball with my dad and sister, roughhoused with my cousins, and felt strong enough to go to school. And that's what the Hannahs did as well. They thanked God for blessing them with a healthy son. Because of their focus, Danielle and Casey were able to keep climbing, and on August 15, 2019, Danielle gave birth to a beautiful little girl named Callie, and on June 23, 2021, Danielle and Casey welcomed another blessing to their family—Luke Isaac.

I'm so thankful I mastered this mountain technique at a young age. It helped me climb, and the more I climbed, the more I understood something. If the right tools aren't in my backpack, then like a sudden and unexpected gust of wind, the climb becomes dangerous.

MOUNTAIN GUIDE TO THE NEXT PEAK:

1. What losses have you experienced in life?
2. List some of your *cans* and *joys* in your life.
3. In addition to focusing on the *cans* and *joys* in your life, what other ways can you pre-acclimate so you can keep climbing?

_____

_____

_____

_____

_____

_____

_____

_____

_____

_____

_____

_____

_____

_____

_____

_____

_____

_____

NOT IN MY BACKPACK

There are far better things ahead than the ones we leave behind. —C.S. Lewis

I couldn't take it anymore, and I was done.

No one should be expected to take this much medicine—small chalky pills dissolved with the littlest bit of moisture, giant horse pills, and liquid so bitter it set my throat on fire.

Mornings became a dreaded routine.

"Whitney, you can't get up until you've taken all of your medicine," my parents would say. My will was much stronger than my parents, and most mornings, I sat for hours with one parent who coaxed me to take each pill—one by one.

One day, my little eight-year-old mind formulated a plan. *I can pour my cup of juice with medicine out, wrap my pills in a napkin, stuff the napkin in the cup, and throw it away.* And I did. I knew there were certain pills I needed to take to live, so I continued to take those medications. But the other pills were unnecessary, and into the trash they went.

As strong as my little will was, my conscience was stronger. One evening in church, I decided I must tell my mom. I wrote her a note.

Dear Mom,
I need to confess something to you. For the last two weeks, I have been throwing my medicine away. You

can punish me any way you want, but I hope you're proud of me for being honest.
Love, Whitney

Yes, even at the age of eight, I knew how to pull at heartstrings with my words. I'm sure I got in serious trouble, although now I can't remember the series of events that took place when we arrived home after church. I still chuckle at this memory, and my mom kept the precious note.

At eight, I had yet another bitter pill to swallow, one I could not throw away or hide in a napkin. If God never healed me, then the truth was taking medicine would be something I must do for the rest of my life.

Unfortunately, the difficult and complex issues were only beginning. I learned to wear a brave face. I needed the courage to face cruelty and hostility from the ones I thought were my friends. Don't ever believe someone who tells you the words and actions of others shouldn't have the power to affect you—a harsh lesson I learned at a young age.

One afternoon, my English teacher finished her lecture early and gave us free time. Excitement filled my heart. I had the rare chance to hang and laugh with my friends at school.

"Whitney, you should be in the Guinness Book of World Records for having the most warts." My classmate laughed as if he'd cracked a joke rivaling those on the comedy circuit.

I felt the warmth rush into my cheeks as humiliation and embarrassment stole my joy, exuberance, and contentment. The betrayal overshadowed the security I felt. I considered this boy a friend, and he hurt me in the worst way possible.

My friend threw her arm around my shoulder and railed at him with rage matching her red hair. "How could you say something like that to her?"

I was thankful for her rebuke because I couldn't speak. My grief and pain prevented me from processing a sentence.

"What happened?" another boy asked.

"Oh, he just told Whitney she should be in the Guinness Book of World Records for having the most warts." Sarcasm and annoyance dripped from my friend's words. My feelings were a mixture of thankfulness and frustration. I was grateful my friend was still angry about what happened and for her support of me, but I worried the hurtful and unnecessary dig would spread like wildfire as most drama did with kids.

His eyes grew round, and he laughed an uncomfortable and shocked laugh—disbelief someone was so cruel to me but amused by the joke.

Who else will they tell? These words chipped away at my confidence.

I had undergone extensive wart surgeries in the past, where the blemishes were cut and burned, and I was wrapped from head to toe with gauze, like a burn patient. I hoped the pain I put myself through would prevent the warts from coming back, and beautiful skin would take their place. But alas, the disease raging in my body generated warts, and the steroids I was on for my weakened immune system fed them. My clothes became my human shield to hide what I didn't want to be seen, but they didn't cover the blemishes on my face. After choosing to accept I needed medication, I didn't expect to be a dartboard for my peer's malicious and brazen comments.

The disease was on the warpath to see what it could destroy. It set its sights on my sinuses and bones. Sinus infection after sinus infection led to multiple sinus surgeries, and with the help of long-term steroid usage, my disease chipped away at my bones. My immune system thrived on steroids, but my bones and joints were beaten to a pulp by the medication known as a double-edged sword. The steroids caused a disease in my bones called *avascular necrosis*.

Avascular necrosis eats away at the bone and the cartilage between bones to the point the bone collapses, and the cartilage disappears. This caused my knees to buckle, catch, and in the scariest, most severe episodes, hyperextend and lock to where I couldn't move. Orthopedic surgery to remove the floating pieces of cartilage was the answer.

These surgeries led to permanent scarring and accented my warts. I didn't feel I fit the mold of what society deemed normal and attractive. I felt exposed, vulnerable, and unattractive. The feeling of free-falling with nothing to grasp to gain steadiness was the most helpless feeling. I couldn't choose to stop my medication, so the warts returned after surgery, and I couldn't refuse to undergo surgery if I wanted the best quality of life. I was at the mercy of my disease and others' cruelty, and the feeling of helplessness was miserable.

How does one climb with the excess weight of weakness?

When a climber prepares to ascend a mountain, they are obsessed with making their load as light as possible. With good reason, because climbing a mountain takes endurance and perseverance. Unnecessary weight will slow a climber, produce exhaustion, and drain their strength. This can lead to dangerous situations for a climber. Even the recommended list of essentials is lengthy. Some pieces of equipment are dependent on what type of mountain a person's climbing—you don't need tools for ice if you're rock climbing, but the purpose of a checklist is to help the climber choose the appropriate types and amounts of supplies and equipment. A mountain climber may need to research and decide what is essential to put in their backpack for the mountain they are climbing.

The important question at hand is what do I need in my backpack, and what will be an unnecessary burden? Here are just some of the recommendations from *wikiHow*'s article, "How to Climb a Mountain." A mountain climber will need to consider: warm clothing, climbing boots with crampons, ice ax and hammer, helmet, harness, gaiters, harness, belay break, head lamb, lightweight backpack, ropes and carabiners, tape for abseil loops, ice screws, nuts, slings, small first aid kit, sunscreen, lip salve, sunglasses, goggles, tent to withstands weather, sleeping bag, cooking supplies, food, water, straw, small pocket knife, feces and urine removal kit and loo paper, climbing permit, map, compass/GPS, camera, and passport (if crossing borders).[1]

See why experts stress vanity and materialistic items must be left behind? Anything more than what's needed will be a burden and a hindrance.

Remember how I said not to ever believe anyone who tells you another's words and actions shouldn't have the power to affect you? They indeed will, and that's okay. You're human, and you're allowed to feel and react to the hurt others cause you. But it's how you move forward with the hurt and pain that matters. That's how you gain control despite the actions of others you can't control. The weight of some emotions and hurt can take longer to shed. The first step is to know what to take out of your backpack so you can make it to the top of your mountain.

The more I removed unhealthy or false perceptions of myself, the higher I ascended on my mountain. I could either choose to see my medication as confining or accept the side effects and move on to something I enjoyed. I could either detest the scars my surgeries caused or look at them as beautiful reminders of what I'd overcome and a sign of my strength. I could either allow the hurtful comments my classmates uttered about my warts to warp my self-image, or I could accept the truth my warts didn't take away from my beauty. The more I released this negativity, the clearer my views became.

If you've already taken to heart what has been done or said to you, it's not too late to take the negative out of your backpack and replace it with the beautiful truths of how God sees you. He sees the beautiful soul he knitted within you. He knows your innermost strengths, dreams, and talents. He knows you are a mountain warrior, and you are MORE than capable of conquering the sharp and insurmountable cliffs and terrain you face. Just as he always saw those truths in me, he saw it in my sister.

Last September, I had the honor of hosting my sister, Linsay, on *Mountain Climbers*. My bubbly and energetic sister always worried about what others thought of her. Confrontation put her stomach in knots, and when something didn't go as planned, she would go into panic mode. Finally, when the nervousness affected her health, she decided to see a doctor and was diagnosed with anxiety.

"It was just this snowball effect. I had shingles three times around my eye in four months, and I was on blood pressure medicine. It's been hard to admit, and I struggled coming forward and being vulnerable with it because I was afraid people would view me as less than Christian," Linsay shared.

But Linsay realized being ashamed of her internal struggle and the stigma of anxiety in the world, even in the church world, was not something she should believe or hide behind anymore.

"My nurse practitioner looked at me and said, 'I'm first going to tell you your faith is intact, and you're not weak for needing help and medication.' I needed to hear that because I knew I couldn't go on as I was anymore," my sister said through her tears.

Linsay's nurse practitioner referred her to a Christian counselor and prescribed medication.

Linsay read Scripture, exercised, and got enough sleep. When she removed the angst from her backpack, the pressure and weight on her heart and soul lifted. With the weight gone, she was able to fill her backpack with truthful and empowering beliefs such as confidence, assurance, and contentment, which led her to climb higher. She saw the mountaintop views God had for her—as well as new friendships, a new home, marriage, and motherhood.

Just as climbers need their backpacks to store what is essential for their climb, we need our spiritual backpack filled with what's important for life's mountains.

Philippians 4:8 tells us to think about things that are true, honest, just, pure, lovely, and of a good report. And those attitudes are what we need in our backpacks to climb to the top and make our souls feel light and joyous. The possibility of a beautiful new peak is just on the horizon.

MOUNTAIN GUIDE TO THE NEXT PEAK:

1. What unpleasant tasks must you do to be a healthy and well-rounded person?
2. Has someone ever said something cruel or hurtful to you? How did it make you feel?
3. If you believed them, how can you lighten your backpack so you can keep climbing?
4. How do you think God sees you? List some attributes which are true, honest, just, pure, lovely, and of a good report to put in your backpack.

_____

_____

_____

_____

_____

_____

_____

_____

_____

_____

_____

_____

_____

_____

_____

_____

_____

_____

_____

THE BRIDGE TO THE RIDGE

Faith is the bridge between where I am and the place where God is taking me. —Unknown

"How's Whitney?" Dr. M asked my mom. The more my disease progressed, the more he realized my disease's major components were autoimmune and immune issues. Dr. M made the difficult decision to pass my care over to the hematology department.

As they sat in his office, my mom squirmed in her seat. This was the open door she prayed for, but how does one tell a doctor one of their colleagues was neglectful without sounding overly critical?

"Whitney is doing okay. She's always fragile, but for right now, she's stable with high doses of steroids. But honestly, we haven't had the best experience with her hematologists. They tried a new treatment called *intravenous immune globulin therapy* (IVIg) made from the antibodies of donated plasma. Whitney responded to it well. But then there was a shortage of donations, and she couldn't receive it anymore. Her hematologists sent us home with Whitney on high doses of steroids, telling us to give them some time to come up with a treatment plan, and they would call." Mom sighed. "That was nine months ago."

His eyes darkened, and his cheeks reddened. "Mrs. Ward, you mean to tell me they have left Whitney unmonitored for nine months on steroids without an appointment or even a phone call to see how she is doing?"

The lines etched on my mom's face were a testament to her frustration and exhaustion. "Yes. I know Whitney's case is complicated, but the one thing her father and I requested was we didn't want her to remain on steroids because of the long-term effects on her body. And now she's been on them for almost a year. I don't want it to seem like I'm bad-mouthing another doctor to you, but I know this can't be safe. My husband and I are at a loss at what to do, but one thing we do know is our daughter needs and deserves better care."

Dr. M held his hand up in comfort and understanding. "Please do not worry, Mrs. Ward. I agree this is too long for Whitney to be on this dose of steroids. I'm sorry I was unaware. At the end of this appointment, we're going to make another appointment for Whitney with me."

My mom could barely hold back her tears. "Thank you. This is exactly what I've prayed for."

I was so excited to have my beloved doctor back. Once again, he became the guide my parents and I needed. Yes, my case was complicated, but he was willing to do something my hematologists were not. He tried to help me. He pushed his rheumatology expertise to the max, trying to fill the role of three doctors, rheumatology, hematology, and immunology.

Although still innocent, I had developed a keen understanding of how to listen to my body at a young age, but I didn't understand how crucial it was to have a doctor trained to treat autoimmune and immune diseases. My parents understood this, and they prayed for a bridge. That bridge came in the form of my uncle, James, but first, my uncle needed to relocate.

James was married to my dad's sister, Aunt Leslie, and he was a pharmaceutical representative. He and my aunt lived in Georgia, the state where my dad grew up. They loved living in Georgia. They were close to family and were involved in their church. They had no intention of ever leaving their community—until James' pharmaceutical company transferred him to North Carolina. My aunt and uncle experienced confusion, anger, fear, and insecurity. They were about to leave the security and harness of what they knew.

At times, during a climb to the summit, one vital piece of equipment a climber will need is a climbing harness. Tim Peck and Doug Martland share in an article on *goEast*, that a harness secures a person to their rope, anchoring the climber to the mountain. A harness must be functionally safe and comfortable. Why? Because when you fall or want to take a break from climbing, the harness is what secures you to your rope in case of a fall and can also become a seat. This comfort is essential so a climber can make it to the top of the summit.[1]

But for life's mountains, sometimes the security of a harness can also hinder our climb. My uncle didn't understand why God was asking him to remove his harness and relocate for his job, but it soon became clear it wasn't just for him. God wanted James to be a catalyst to help me.

Ring! Ring! Ring! "Hello?" Dad answered our black rotary phone.

"Hey, Brent, this is James."

"Hey, buddy! How are you?"

"I'm good. How are Cathy and the girls?"

"They are good. I can't complain at all. How's everybody in your neck of the woods?"

"We're doing good as well. Listen, the reason for my call is to discuss something that involves Whitney. One of my clients is Duke University. The hematology department, actually, and I've developed a good relationship with one of the hematologists."

"Wow." Dad chuckled. "Are you serious?"

"Yes. I hope I haven't overstepped, but I've talked to her about Whitney and how mysterious her illness is. She's very interested in Whitney's case and would like to see her. Do you think this is something you and Cathy would be interested in for Whitney?"

"Oh wow, buddy, you didn't overstep. This is an answer to our prayers. As you know, we're in very uncertain times with Whitney's health. We love Whitney's rheumatologist. He's a Godsend, but he's not the type of specialist she needs. Let me talk to Cathy, but I'd say we're very much on board with this. I can't thank you enough for thinking of Whitney."

My parents were ecstatic. Out of respect, my mom called my rheumatologist and asked what he thought about this opportunity. He urged my parents to take me to the prestigious hospital.

It was a lot for a ten-year-old to process. But excitement overrode every emotion as I was embarking on a grand adventure to North Carolina. I'd get to see family, and I'd gained the interest of another doctor who could discover what was wrong with me. Above all, I still had the comfort and security of my rheumatologist, Dr. M. He approved this trip, so that gave me peace of mind.

I was in awe of Duke University and its caliber. The best description is it is like watching a grade-school musical and then seeing the same musical on Broadway. The wonder of the special effects and costumes is a sight to behold. The lights are brighter, and the costumes more realistic. Duke University was a medical Broadway show.

My uncle accompanied my parents and me from department to department, providing a comforting presence in yet another new medical world. I'd never had so much blood taken from my little veins.

"Honey, you can't walk. Just look at all those tubes I took from you, you tiny thing—no walking for you. Your daddy is going to need to carry you," the kind phlebotomist told me as she showered me with apple juice and graham crackers.

I clicked with the young hematologist as I had with my rheumatologist and responded to her warmth. Just as the line of doctors who came to feel my enlarged spleen during my first visit at Cincinnati Children's, doctors at Duke came to feel my infamously large organ. My new hematologist had an astounding thought about this thorn in my side. Remove it!

"Not only is the organ diseased, but it could be what's causing her illness." She surmised while prodding my left side. "But before we set Whitney up with our surgery department, I want immunology to weigh in. I know immunologists are more lab-oriented than clinical, and that's why Whitney doesn't have one. But since the other major component to Whitney's disease is immunological and we have clinical immunologists at Duke, I feel it's crucial to get them to consult."

Although nervous about another major surgery, I also felt eager—a world of new opportunities awaited on the other side. My new doctor's instinct to consult with immunology proved to be one of amazing insight.

"No, don't remove her spleen. The spleen and liver share a lot of the same functions. If the spleen is removed, there's a chance whatever is wrong with her spleen could transfer over to the liver. That would be detrimental," the immunologist declared with voice low and eyes wide. "She can live without a spleen, but she can't live without a liver."

In my mind, the trip and new doctors didn't change my life much. I thought it was a cool experience, but I wouldn't be having surgery, and my doctors at Duke didn't make any discoveries. But, to me, that had been the whole point of the trip. I had no clue my world was about to be turned upside down.

"Mr. and Mrs. Ward, I would love to be Whitney's hematologist, but with how much care she needs, it's not practical with you living in Ohio." My hematologist leaned forward. "But in my most sincere and strongest medical opinion, Whitney cannot go back to Cincinnati's hematology department. Her health will worsen with the lack of care she received. I want to suggest Columbus Children's Hospital. Whitney's main doctor needs to be a hematologist. There is a hematologist there I have the utmost respect for and confidence in his ability. His name is Dr. Randal Olshefski. Is this something you would consider? If so, I'll make the referral."

My parents looked at each other.

"Yes, we'd consider it." My dad spoke first.

"Whitney's rheumatologist at Cincinnati has been so kind, going above and beyond for Whitney. I'm sure he'll be on board with this and do what he needs to do to transfer her care, but out of respect for all he's done for our daughter, I want to speak to him before we give our final answer." Mom said.

As I listened to this conversation, I didn't worry. I believed he would want to keep me as a patient.

Later, I sat in my uncle's kitchen, listening to my mom talk to my doctor.

"What do you think, Dr. M?"

Silence.

"Are you sure? We will stay with you if you feel like that's what we should do."

No! I strained to hear the rest of the conversation.

"Well, I want you to know." Mom's voice cracked. "I want you to know how much my husband and I appreciate everything you have done for Whitney. We will never forget it." Mom sobbed.

No, this can't be happening!

"Mom! I don't want to leave him!"

"Sweetie, I know. I don't want to leave him either. But we have no choice. You have to have a hematologist, and we can't go back to Cincinnati."

I didn't say much else. I took it like I did every punch in the gut. I grieved silently. I didn't understand it then, but I removed the harness to inch closer to my summit.

My assistant pastor and *Mountain Climbers* guest, Brian Baer, understands what it takes to remove the harness of comfort zones. Brian grew up attending Beech Fork Church in the area called Otway, Ohio. His family was involved in the church, and everyone assumed Brian would become a leader in his home church, maybe even pastor it someday. But after serving as the evangelist for Rubyville Community Church's youth camp, God asked Brian to remove his harness attached to the security at Beech Fork Church and move his family to Rubyville Community Church.

"It was in 2004 when that feeling started to come. It was like ... I can't explain it, just a sense of you're not complete."

Even though Brian knew this move was what God was calling him to do, he still struggled with what others would think, especially his family.

"I wasn't going to Rubyville to be an assistant pastor or a youth leader. I was going just to go. It went against everything I had been taught. You don't leave a good church just to go to another good church." Brian shared.

"It was the toughest decision I ever made. I didn't want to leave my mom and dad. I didn't want to leave my papaw, who was one of my heroes. I didn't want to disappoint my family." Brian choked through the tears. "When you're used to something, and you're comfortable, and you're still being used ... man, it was just so tough."

But even though the calling didn't make sense, Brian took off his harness and left the certainty of what he knew to climb toward the top of his mountain, which was assistant pastor of Rubyville Community Church.

"In 2006, when it happened, and I became assistant pastor, for the first time in my life, I felt like I had arrived." Brian beamed.

My young heart didn't know it yet, but when I took off my secure and comfortable harness to meet my new hematologist, Dr. Olshefski, I had arrived, just like Brian. My Uncle James was willing to take off his harness and be a bridge for me, so I could take off mine.

As mountain climbers, we should strive to know when to remove our harnesses and be a bridge for others. What an honor to connect them to their purpose. In doing so, God can take us to new heights and maybe even bring some new teammates for the climb.

IN LOVING MEMORY OF JAMES COMPTON
BELOVED HUSBAND, FATHER, GRANDFATHER,
UNCLE, AND BRIDGE.

Mountain Guide to the Next Peak:

1. Can you think of a time you were in a predicament and didn't know how to handle it? How did God make a way for you?
2. Name someone who was a bridge for you, connecting you from one season of your life to the next season.
3. How can you be a bridge for someone in your life?
4. Do you have a harness in your life you need to step out of? What can you do to leave your comfort zone and climb to the purpose God has for you?

_____

_____

_____

_____

_____

_____

_____

_____

_____

_____

_____

_____

_____

_____

_____

_____

_____

_____

A NEW TEAM

Alone we can do so little, together we can do so much.
—Helen Keller

My mom and I watched the doctor walk in—her skirt and *clickety-clack* of heels stated the obvious—this was not Dr. Olshefski. My mother's eyes widened, and her mouth dropped. I thought she might fall out of her chair.

"I'm so sorry for my reaction, but my daughter is supposed to see Dr. Olshefski."

"Oh, I apologize. There must have been a mix-up." The doctor offered a half-smile, clearly embarrassed."

"Listen, I'm sure you're a good doctor. I don't want it to seem like I'm overreacting, but my daughter's care has been unpredictable and uncertain the last year." Mom took a deep breath. "We didn't have a good experience at her previous hospital. Her hematologist at Duke specifically wanted us to see Dr. Olshefski and made the referral. I have to fight for my daughter's care, and he's who my husband and I want her to see."

I squirmed in my seat—I hated confrontation and awkwardness.

The doctor lowered her head, showing her graciousness and humbleness. "I understand, Mrs. Ward. You must do what you feel is best for your child. We will make an appointment with Dr. Olshefski on your way out."

My mom was an amazing advocate, teaching me to listen to my gut and instincts. Her example taught me how to advocate for myself as an adult, expecting nothing but the best care from my physicians. But I love this moment because it's the first time I recognized and understood the lengths she would go to make sure the specialists showed me compassion and cared for me as a person and not just a *medical case*. I had no way of knowing at the time, but my mother's insistence that Dr. Olshefski be my hematologist was a turning point for my medical care. Each visit and encounter with the doctor, it became more and more evident God was the orchestrator of my care. Dr. Olshefski had no idea what autoimmune disease he was dealing with, and yet, he had a keen instinct and wisdom for what my body needed and would respond to.

He weaned me off steroids, understanding this potent but destructive drug wasn't a permanent solution. To counteract the boost my body lost due to the steroid weaning, I started the IVIg therapy to counteract the loss of steroid treatments. My low immune system took to the new treatment like milk and honey.

But aside from being in tune with what my body needed, Dr. Olshefski did something else critical. It's what separates the good doctors from the great ones—he took the time to foster a relationship with me. I wasn't just a case to him, I was a person, and that resonated with me.

If you know me, you know I'm fluent in sarcasm and snark. There wasn't an appointment that Dr. Olshefski and I didn't try to one-up each other with a zanier one-liner.

My mom, ever the organized teacher, had one request with each appointment—I wear clean socks with no holes. It took two hours to get from my home to Columbus Children's Hospital, now known as Nationwide Children's Hospital. Without fail, five minutes before we arrived, my mom would look in the rearview mirror, catch my eye, and ask if I had clean socks without holes. One day, she didn't ask her standard one-liner, and I was glad because I had ignored her biggest pet peeve.

"Okay, Whitney, take your shoes off and let me see your feet." Dr. Olshefski said.

The moment had arrived. I took my shoes off, bracing myself for the reveal that the hole in my sock was as big as the eye could see.

Mom put her head in her hand. "Whitney Lane." Then she looked up at the doctor. "Dr. Olshefski, I'm sorry. I promise I try to make sure she puts on decent socks before we leave the house."

Dr. Olshefski grinned and took his shoe off. "It's okay. I have a hole in my sock today too."

He's the essence of what a doctor should be. Someone who becomes relatable to their patients, coming to where they are. Being immersed in the world of sickness and disease is scary for anyone of any age, but for a child trying to understand why they are scared and process the complex reasons, it is even scarier. Dr. Olshefski created a secure and safe feeling in the midst of an ever-changing and overwhelming world. It was okay I didn't understand it all because he didn't either—but he worked hard to understand my Rubik's cube of an immune system. The most profound knowledge Dr. Olshefski possessed was this—he couldn't do it alone.

There are many rules for mountain climbing, and *wikiHow* stresses one of monumental importance—never climb a mountain alone. Climbing a mountain takes strength and stamina, not only mentally but physically. Climbers need to depend on each other and problem-solve together. One climber may be an excellent navigator, while another climber may be able to spot the perfect foothold to advance the team to the summit. Everyone has strengths and weaknesses, and what one climber may excel at, another mountaineer may not. Success and survival depend on teamwork and each climber having the other's back.[1]

Another major reason climbing alone isn't recommended is because a climber depends on another person known as the belayer. *Sportrock*, a climbing center in Alexandria, Virginia, explains a belayer's job is to hold the end of the rope attached to the climber's harness, pulling it tight when the climber falls, protecting them from plunging downward.[2]

Dr. Olshefski understood my disease was multi-faceted. His expertise was in my hematological issues. For my other medical abnormalities, he needed to recruit new team members—medical *belayers*. The first new team member was my new rheumatologist. Again, I gained a new doctor I clicked with. Each visit, before she asked questions about my condition, we discussed the hobby I was most passionate about—reading. My new rheumatologist, Dr. Gloria Higgins, was impressed and fascinated that my nose was stuck in a book every time she came into my room. We discussed what I was reading, and she always wanted to know what each book was about. Again, she was a doctor who came to where I was and related to me as a human being.

However, I was about to discover that even if I didn't click right away with one of my doctors, it didn't mean they weren't a valuable player. They each could become an MVP.

"I really need an immunologist on Whitney's case." Dr. Olshefski told my mother and me during one appointment. "We don't have one here yet, but we are getting one soon. When he gets here, can I set her up with an appointment with him?"

"Of course, whatever you think Whitney needs, we are on board with," My mom told him.

Several months later, I sat in an exam room waiting for my immunologist, Dr. P, to walk through the door. With little introduction, I soon realized this man was every inch a scientist with his critical mind already working on angles of why my immune system was such a mystery. When I cracked a joke, and his face was blank, I knew we had a long way to go to understand each other. But his nurse practitioner would always laugh, so that broke the ice.

What I didn't count on was a doctor who had a phobia with feet. With each visit, he asked me if he could see my feet. Then he would stand as far back as propriety would allow with his hands behind his back. I felt as my feet were a freak of nature, and with each visit, I got more and more annoyed.

One day, he asked his standard question, "Uhh, Whitney, can I see your feet?" Fighting the urge to roll my eyes, I turned my back to him to take my shoes and socks off. What I didn't know was that, for the first time since he became my doctor, he was standing right behind me to look at my feet. I took one shoe and sock off without a hitch. Then I took my other shoe off and found my sock was stuck. I tugged and tugged. Finally, it flew off and made perfect contact with D. P's face. I turned to hide my smile. His round eyes showed his shock and disgust. My nurse practitioner giggled, and my mother's expression told everyone she wished she could disappear through the floor.

As I got older, I saw a change in Dr. P. I became a person to him and not just a complicated medical case for him to decipher. Even though our senses of humor were on opposite sides of the spectrum, I knew he cared about me. The prophylactic antibiotics he put me on were just what my body needed, and he was always researching and looking for possibilities of new medications and treatments to strengthen my weak immune system.

A couple of years after Dr. P became my doctor, it became clear God had a plan beyond anyone's imagination when I discovered Dr. P had done his fellowship at Duke University. His teacher was the immunologist I saw when I was a patient there, and Dr. P's fellowship took place at the same time I was there. It was evident to me God orchestrated something miraculous with my team of doctors, and his infinite and beautiful plan was unfolding, but I wouldn't know the whole purpose for years to come. What I did know was this—Dr. Olshefski, Dr. P, Dr. Higgins, and later, Dr. Stacey Ardoin, who became my rheumatologist after Dr. Higgins retired, went above and beyond investing in me not just as a patient, but as a person who had hopes and dreams. Dr. Ardoin championed and supported my writing and found ways I could speak at events and share my story. It was clear these were the doctors God had chosen for me. In time, this would become evident to all.

This is what it takes for anyone to climb life's mountains—a team. It may be our mountain to face, but we can't make it alone. We, of course, need God's strength, but in his infinite wisdom, God GIVES us teammates for life. Parents, grandparents, siblings, friends, pastors, teachers, and of course, doctors and nurses—people God knows will give us our perfect assist to help us be victorious. These people pray for us, give us godly wisdom, encourage us, and heal our wounds, whether physical or invisible.

If anyone knows what it means to be on a team, it's my *Mountain Climbers'* guest, Shanae Cruse. The trail she had to take to get there is nothing short of heartbreaking. Shanae was a basketball star with so much talent, the great Pat Summit recruited her. But her skill and the prestige of being recognized for her gift went to her head.

"When you come from a small town where basketball is everything, and you're good at it, people tend to give you some slack. When you have a D or an F, and you really shouldn't be playing, or if you want to skip out on class, people kind of afford you luxuries just because you are a good basketball player." Shanae explained. And she thrived on these luxuries. "Unfortunately, I got a big head to the point I would sign autographs. I would tell people that I would be famous one day, so you better keep this. I became a person you wouldn't like."

One fateful night, Shanae experienced the nightmare no athlete wants to face when she tore her ACL during a game.

What Shanae didn't know at the time was God allowed this to happen so she could be a part of a team with an eternal impact. "I began a very long journey of recovery, and that's when I realized my identity was in the wrong things. It made me open my eyes to who I identified with and what I identified in."

This was the turning point for Shanae, and she allowed God to shift her focus. She realized when she put her identity in Christ, she was more than just a basketball player. "I ended up at my home church, and I told God I wanted to be all in and asked what that looked like. I wanted to become a member. I wanted to tithe. I wanted to be a part of a small group. A part of being a member is you have to serve, and I said, okay, I'll serve with students. I'm not too old yet. I can hang out with kids," she said with a laugh.

Every Wednesday night, Shanae led a small group of teen girls she could pour herself into and still does life with to this day. "What I came to realize serving with this group is they need someone to tell them what God says they are and not what the world does. And so, I found my place to help and hopefully allow God to use me, so someone didn't go down the same route I did," Shanae shared with conviction.

We make it to the top of our mountains by realizing we can't do it alone and need to utilize the teammates God gives us. We take on the responsibility of helping our teammates climb to the top of their mountains as well. The book of Ephesians explains—we all make a body. God gives every one of his children gifts and abilities, so we can all work together to achieve the highest summits. Here's the most important truth of why you need your team by your side—because with every mountain comes unexpected cliffs and uneven terrain.

MOUNTAIN GUIDE TO THE NEXT PEAK:

1. Why is it important you advocate for yourself to have who you need to climb the mountain?
2. Who are your teammates? How have they helped you climb?
3. What are your gifts and abilities God has given you? How can you help others climb their mountains?

_____

_____

_____

_____

_____

_____

_____

_____

_____

_____

_____

_____

_____

_____

_____

_____

_____

_____

_____

A NORMAL JOURNEY

The comeback is always stronger than the setback. —
Unknown.

My sister and I giggled as we walked out to surprise our
parents. They had gone to a Valentine's Day party at their
friend's house, and Linsay and I spent the evening with
our grandparents.

"Get those off!" my dad screeched in horror when he saw
what we were wearing. He didn't like seeing his daughters
in wedding dresses and picturing us all grown up with
husbands. My dad was a girl-dad through and through, and
we, his daughters, had him wrapped around our little fingers.

We were donned in all white. I wore my mother's wedding
dress, and my sister wore my aunt's. All the women in his
life howled in merriment over my dad's reaction, and my
grandma ran for the camera. Linsay and I thrived on the
attention and struck a pose.

"Ow!" A fiery hot pain shot through my left side.

"Are you okay, Sis?" My mom asked.

"Yeah. My side had a pain in it, but it's gone now."

"Ok, well, keep an eye on it and let me know if it hurts
again."

"Okay, I will."

A couple of weeks later, I was in church. My pastor
asked all the youth to come to the front to be recognized.

It is amazing how one second a person can be fine, and the next moment their life changes forever. I walked up with my friends, feeling good and appreciative that my pastor was encouraging our church's youth. Then, a few minutes later, the sharp, fiery darts of pain shot through the left side again. This time, they were more intense.

I walked back to my parents' pew in tears. "My spleen is hurting." I choked out. My mom and dad guided me down the aisle. Even amid my pain, I could see the concern on people's faces as they noticed the tears streaming down my face.

My parents laid me on the floor in a Sunday school room. Fear and panic were etched in their wide eyes and lowered brows.

My mother pleaded with my father, "Brent, we need to do something! Pray!"

My dad prayed God would take away my pain. And he did take the edge off to where I could go home, but it was clear my body was trying to tell me something was wrong. A couple of days later, my mom and I sat with Dr. Olshefski. He told us my spleen was inflamed. The next few days would go in one direction—the inflammation would ease, or my infamous organ would die. Over the next few days, my body gave the answer. The diseased organ began a slow and painful death. A CAT scan showed my spleen was experiencing an infarction, a strange medical term meaning my organ's blood was clotting and losing its circulation— my spleen was dying.

My Achilles heel of a spleen took so much from me. This season of new medical developments was scary, painful, and exhausting. The comfort of the consistent unknowns and my doctor's blind treatment of an undiagnosed disease became a sense of security. Amid all the unanswered questions, I came to know what to expect. Now I was embarking on a whole different level—filled with unknown territories. But in the depths of my soul, I wondered if this was the beginning of some normalcy? Would I get to experience any sort of a carefree childhood?

My surgery was scheduled ASAP. My ambitious surgeon even agreed to do three surgeries in one, not only removing my spleen but also my gall bladder and another crop of warts. It was obvious to everyone this would not be a minor surgery. Amid it all, my parents tried to make the situation a little less frightening by keeping a sense of routine and familiarity, so the night before my surgery, we headed to Columbus and stayed in a hotel just as we did for every sinus surgery and ear tube placement. This tradition softened the dread and anxiety of surgery by eliminating a long car ride the morning of the procedure.

The mix of relief and fear was intertwined. Relief the pain would be gone, and fear of being cut into in a new and major way. I woke that morning with acceptance of what I would face and realized I couldn't breathe. The pain was intense. Each breath I took felt like a bowling ball hitting a strike between my two lungs, which added to the dread of the unknown I was about to face. Before my family and I left the hotel to head to the hospital, Dad gathered us around to read Scripture. He chose to read Psalm 23.

> The Lord is my shepherd; I shall not want. He maketh me to lie down in green pastures: he leadeth me beside the still waters. He restoreth my soul: he leadeth me in the paths of righteousness for his name's sake. Yea, though I walk through the valley of the shadow of death.

Sobs wracked my dad's body, and tears streamed down my mom's and sister's cheeks. The enormity of the situation had finally overpowered them.

What did I do? I took the Bible from my dad and continued reading.

> Yea, though I walk through the valley of the shadow of death, I will fear no evil: for thou art with me; thy

rod and thy staff they comfort me. Thou preparest a table before me in the presence of mine enemies: thou anointest my head with oil; my cup runneth over. Surely goodness and mercy shall follow me all the days of my life: and I will dwell in the house of the LORD for ever.

Dad didn't know it then—I didn't even know it right then, but at that moment, he taught me how powerful Scripture is. In an ever-changing world, God's Word would remain constant and give a sense of peace to calm even my most anxious soul. When the surgical team wheeled me away from my parents, the numbness disappeared, and stark fear replaced it. Tears rained down my face, and the well-meaning nurse tried to soothe my terror by telling me it was all going to be okay. I wondered if she realized how empty and clichéd her reassurance sounded. She wasn't the one lying on the gurney. As the surgical team rolled my bed closer to the OR, the Holy Spirit whispered to my heart what would calm any fear and anxiety—I quoted Scripture. Over and over, I said my favorite verse, Isaiah 41:10: "Fear thou not; for I am with thee: be not dismayed; for I am thy God: I will strengthen thee; yea, I will help thee; yea, I will uphold thee with the right hand of my righteousness." The tears still flowed, but the overwhelming terror that threatened to suffocate me subsided, and peace took its place.

Later, I woke from a successful surgery and found out my spleen had had one final ace up its sleeve. It had attached itself to my diaphragm, hence the extreme pain and difficulty breathing. I recovered, and a strange occurrence happened to my body. I gained new strength and stamina—I felt ... healthy. I had my first post-check-up with Dr. Olshefski, and I found out the reason. For the first time in my life, my blood counts were normal.

"Well, I've got some good news for you both. Whitney's blood counts are normal." Dr. Olshefski shared with a smile.

"Really?" I exclaimed, my body jolting with excitement.

"What's this mean?" My mom asked with caution and hope mingled in her voice.

My specialist shrugged in surprised happiness. "Based on her lab results and how well she is doing, I'd say her spleen was causing her disease. She's now in remission. I don't need to see her for another six months, and then if her counts are still normal, we can go to yearly appointments."

Mom and I grinned at each other. These were words neither of us thought we would ever hear. The next six weeks were idyllic. Nothing could stop me, and I bounced off the walls with activity and had no worry of getting sick or rupturing my spleen. I lost a couple of pant sizes because the enlarged organ no longer bloated my stomach. I had embarked on an exciting new normal life journey.

Isn't that something we all want? Normal. A life with few heartaches and unexpected twists and turns. That's what every mountain climber wants as well—safety, no accidents, and no falls that could lead to a serious injury. And when climbers train and hone their skill as mountaineers, they study mountain climbing rules and regulations and research the mountain they plan on climbing—this preparation will strengthen reactions and quicken critical thinking while high toward the summit. But the possibility of detrimental and life-threatening surprises isn't eliminated, which was something I learned swiftly and devastatingly.

One Sunday morning, six weeks after I had my joyous appointment with my hematologist, I awoke feeling strange. Nausea's fist gripped my stomach. Something was not right with my body. I got out of bed and shuffled to find my mom.

"Hey, Mom, I don't feel good. I think I'm going to vomit."

"It's probably just drainage from your sinuses, sweetie. Eat something and try to get ready for church. You'll probably feel better once you get something on your stomach."

I did as I was told, feeling worse with each passing minute. I managed to get my church clothes on and walked to the bathroom to brush my teeth. But I never got to the sink.

"Mom, Dad! Whitney is vomiting!" My sister called out to our parents.

Bent over the toilet, I looked at my parents standing in the doorway—with ashen and white complexions, they whispered to each other. I was overcome with fatigue and barely able to walk as Mom led me to the couch. All I could think was I needed to rest. I was still in a dress and didn't care. My cousin, a nurse, came over after the church service and confirmed what my parents feared—I was jaundiced.

The next day, Dr. Olshefski confirmed the worse. My hemoglobin had dropped, and I needed to be hospitalized. The removal of my dead, diseased organ shocked my body into a false sense of security. The foreign invader was gone. The truth had now emerged. Eight days of intense monitored high steroid therapy in the hospital, coupled with coming home on high doses of prednisone is what it took to bring my body back to any semblance of stability. Worse than an eight-day hospital stay were the side effects of steroids.

I bloated and was unrecognizable, Dr. Olshefski told me he could put twenty pounds of bricks on my chest, and I wouldn't feel them due to the excessive water weight I now carried. If that weren't enough, the medication caused the warts to thrive again. Not only did all the warts removed during surgery come back, but they had multiplied. The worst part of these unexpected cliffs and terrain I faced was the painful truth I had gotten a taste of what normal was—a glimpse of what a healthy, disease-free body felt like.

In those blissful six weeks, I played ball with no fear that my spleen would rupture. I ran and played games with friends with no worry my body would crash, and I schemed and planned with no thought of being sick when the day of the plans came. Then, in one swift moment, it was all taken away from me. My brief mountaintop victory was gone, and another, bitter, bigger mountain stretched out before me.

Every *Mountain Climbers* guest's quest is unique. They may have climbed similar mountains, but their experiences, perspectives, and stories are all uniquely their own—ones God has given just to them. My cousin LeeAnn Sims, Ben

Cooper, and Michelle Medlock Adams are three people I hosted who have battled cancer. LeeAnn faced ovarian cancer. Ben first battled sinus cancer and then prostate cancer. And Michelle fought melanoma skin cancer. Three similar stories, all authentically their own. But my three guests did have something in common. The mountain came when they least expected it.

LeeAnn, Ben, and Michelle were living life, enjoying God's blessings and gifts, when a mountain erupted from the terrain of their lives and formed with sharp rocks and cliffs. But each of their answers to the mountain was the same—the unknown and unexpected would not make them forget what they knew and could expect—God's faithfulness, promises, and Word.

And that was my answer too. Just as twists and turns come for a mountain climber, when the climb seems to be going according to plan, they must grasp the constant—like their training and research.

It's the same for us climbing life's mountains. My dad laid a foundation the morning of my surgery that took root, and I knew God's Word would remain true and unchangeable—no matter what was before me. I implore you to hide this within your heart as well. Remember what God has done for you in the past, stand on his promises for your future, and prepare to reap those promises of his Word. Then, when you act based on what you know to be true, you will have the strength not to quit just short of your mountaintop victory. When those unmarked trails come your way, you'll be ready to face them with confidence.

MOUNTAIN GUIDE TO THE NEXT PEAK:

1. Looking back, do you recall when an unexpected mountain began for you? What would you have done if you realized your life was about to change forever?
2. What feelings and emotions did you experience when what you considered normal ceased to exist?
3. What truths and promises did you stand on as you climbed an unexpected mountain? What did you learn during that mountain climb that will help you face the next one?

THE UNMARKED TRAIL

Difficult roads lead to beautiful destinations. —Zig
Ziglar

"Wow, he sure is angry." Mom giggled and stated the
obvious about the principal to the school secretary.

Mom signed into the school building, where she spent
most days as booster club president getting the concessions
stand ready for games or organizing fundraisers with
student groups and clubs.

"Well, have a good day. I'm sure I'll see you again."
Mom froze as the principal's door swung open. Filing out
one by one, heads hung low from being scathed by the
tongue lashing they'd received, were several girls from my
class—girls who were supposed to be my friends.

My principal followed them out of his office, still yelling
at the top of his lungs. He glanced over and saw my mom's
wide eyes. "Cathy, I have had it! If they come to me one
more time demanding Whitney doesn't get a gold card or
a blue card or any type of award or recognition, I'll tell
them the next time Whitney is sick or must go to a doctors'
appointment or get a treatment, we'll just switch. They
can go in her place and get her treatment, and Whitney
can come to school and have a day without sickness. It's
absolutely ridiculous, Cathy."

My mom smiled, torn between gratefulness my principal
had stood up for me and the pain of witnessing the hostile

and toxic environment her child encountered when she felt well enough to go to school. My sister's high school experience showed me how competitive those four years could be, but nothing prepared me for what I faced.

What were these girls protesting? A gold, blue, or white card was given to students every nine weeks who received a high GPA and only missed a certain number of days of school during the grading period. This card gave students many perks, including getting into ball games free and being excused from one test for the next nine weeks—and they didn't want me to have one. It broke my heart because, through grade school, my classmates were my friends. They worried about me when I wasn't at school, and I knew they cared about me. They even got me a gift before my splenectomy—I had their support.

My weak immune system and high infection rate caused me to miss seventy-five to one hundred days of school a year, many days over the attendance requirement. My classmates thought my high GPA came from my teachers favoring me, which led to free passes. This belief caused them to feel I didn't deserve the recognition when I wasn't physically in school like them. Their glares and cold shoulders shouted their message and assumptions loud and clear—I wasn't *that* sick, and I was exaggerating my disease to get attention.

I'm so relieved awareness has been raised, and the world has gained empathy for individuals with invisible rare diseases. But when I was in high school, if you didn't have a well-known disease, your authenticity was questioned. Of course, my getting a gold, blue, or white card didn't keep my classmates from receiving one themselves, but they feared this little reward would lead to bigger accolades, like the National Honor Society and scholarships.

What they failed to realize was when I wasn't in school, I had an IEP—an Individualized Education Plan for students with disabilities to lay out accommodations they needed from the school administration to give the students the tools they needed to excel in their education. For example, I worked with a tutor provided by the school, so when I missed school, I had some other type of instruction. When I felt well enough to go to school, my books were left in each classroom so I didn't have to walk back and forth to my locker in between classes and could conserve my energy. Many times, I fell between the cracks with my teachers, and my tutor had to remind them to send home assignments. And during it all, I still completed every assignment, project, quiz, and test the other students in my grade did—often without having the same classroom instruction they had. I did this when I wasn't feeling good, and yet I maintained an excellent GPA. I earned every single grade I was given while facing challenging circumstances. My school's administration believed my efforts should be recognized.

I begged my parents to homeschool me. The toxic, hostile environment became almost unbearable. My parents had to make a tough decision based on what was best for me. "We can't let you run away from confrontation because then you won't know how to face or handle it in the real world."

As an adult, I understand better what they were saying. The treatment I received in high school taught me how important it is to have empathy, compassion, and understanding toward others going through situations I've never experienced. The trail I had to walk was long and painful.

If my classmates saw me doing something enjoyable after I couldn't come to school, they were livid. But there was so much else they didn't see—like how much I had to rest and build my strength to do one fun activity. They didn't understand I didn't have control over when I felt sick and when I felt good enough to enjoy life. If they had understood, they would have known how rare the times were when I had the strength and energy to have a fun outing or exciting activity. And I needed those times so my life would be more than just doctor's appointments and treatments.

My classmates had no clue about the battle I faced every morning when I woke not feeling well, but I strove to go to school. I would make the effort, even if I could only attend for a few hours during the day. The teenagers in my grade didn't see the behind-the-scenes reality. They only saw what they wanted to see.

Since they couldn't persuade my school's administration to withhold recognition I earned fairly, they focused on showing their disdain for me in ways they could control— with hurtful and petty actions.

I always tried to sit in a front-row seat for two reasons—I was hard of hearing, and I was short. In my junior year, almost my entire class had English together, and I chose a front-row seat on the first day of class. I was sick for a few days, and when I came back, another girl had taken my seat in the front row. The only seat left in that row was in the back, and the girl who taken the other seat refused to let me have it back. Crushed doesn't describe what I felt. I walked to the last chair, defeated.

One day, my English teacher walked into the classroom and couldn't find me since I was hidden by other, taller students in front of me. She was a teacher who tried to watch out for me and cared about my well-being.

She looked around the room. "Where's Whitney?"

"She's not here." One girl said, sarcasm dripping from her voice.

My heart thudded in my chest. *Where is this going?*

My teacher leveled her with a look. She was not amused with the girl's attitude or snarky dig. "I know Whitney's here. I just talked to her," she insisted.

"She left early then," the girl responded.

Heat rushed into my cheeks. Did she really just go there?

Humiliated, I raised my hand and waved. "I'm right here."

My teacher shot one more disapproving look at the girl and began her lecture.

In another instance, I walked into my English class and made my way to my back seat. One of the girls in front of me said, "Hey, Whitney, you're here today. How are you doing?"

I was shocked. She cared enough to speak to me and wanted to know how I was. "I'm doing good." I decided to reach out to the empathy I thought I saw in her. "Would I be able to get my seat back?"

The friendly smile faded only to be replaced by distance and annoyance. She reinforced her "no," by telling the other girls to move so the front-row seats would be filled and not by me. I received her message loud and clear—know your place.

My confidence began to crumble, and it showed in the way I carried myself, and I took no pride in my appearance. When I stepped into my high school, I stepped into a suffocating environment with people who told me by their actions I was insignificant, what I had achieved and overcome didn't matter, and my voice shouldn't be heard. I believed them and was determined to stay invisible. I never dared to confess these deepest insecurities because I believed if I admitted I wasn't okay, it would look like I wasn't strong enough to handle my disease. The pain I felt grew, and I hid these deep scars in the depths of my soul for years.

When a mountain climber embarks on a mountain climb, there are many rules and requirements the mountaineer must remember—and one of the biggest measures of safety for them to take to heart is this: Avoid unmarked trails. "Always stay on marked trails. The reasons for this are many. It could be to avoid getting lost or hurt. Unmarked trails often lead to a precipice or other dangerous area," hiker Ryan McClay says. He explained, "It can also be a sign to leave an area alone so it can heal and return to its own natural state." So how does an unmarked trail come to be? "Unmarked trails exist because someone got off the trail to explore. But they rarely actually lead you anywhere you couldn't have gotten to by following the marked trail."

What does a climber do when they've found themselves on an unmarked trail? Ryan explained two options— backtracking to the last known good trail or pressing on, hoping it leads to your destination.

When it comes to life's mountains, for whatever reason, there are times people get off the mountain trail God intended them to climb. When that happens, the answer is to go back to the trail God set your course on. But there are many people who have no control over the unmarked trail they must climb. Here's the good news. God approved the unmarked trail, and it didn't take him by surprise.

The treatment by my peers I faced in high school was my unmarked trail up the mountain. It wasn't something I could control, but I had to trust God had a purpose for this mountain trail to lead me to the destination he intended. How do you climb an unmarked trail? You find purpose. The insecurities and self-doubt that took root in my heart during my teen years would have suffocated me if I'd focused on those feelings and emotions. But God was faithful, and he gave me two passions that helped me climb, passions I still have today—reading and investing in others.

I loved to read. My parents couldn't keep me in books. I loved to read so much my parents would ground me from reading when I got in trouble. Authors like Robin Jones Gunn, Karen Kingsbury, and Lori Wick gave me a safe haven with their words. The characters they created became my friends, and I could escape into their fictional worlds and forget about my reality for a while. I wasn't the insecure sick girl with no self-esteem. I could be anything I wanted to be. It was the exact release I needed to cope with my circumstances. And the countless books I read impacted and strengthened me as a writer.

I also loved investing in others in my youth group at church. I became determined no one I encountered would be made to feel the way I was made to feel. If I could put a smile on someone's face by complimenting them, I would tell them how pretty they looked, or that I liked their outfit. I looked for people who needed a friend and needed to know they mattered, and I showed them they did. Two of the women I reached out to as a teenager are still my dear friends today, and I had the honor of standing with both of them as a bridesmaid when they got married. Investing in others helped take the focus off my problems and gave me a purpose bigger than myself.

Two people who know what it means to climb an unmarked trail are James and Yanissa Cummings, my guests on *Mountain Climbers*. James was diagnosed with Lyme disease. Lyme disease causes inflammation and is a disease transmitted by a parasite, mainly tick bites.

"It really came to a head eight or nine years ago. I started having digestive issues, really bad headaches, and vision issues. It was strange because it just couldn't be pieced together. And every time I would try to nail something down and say this is what it was, then something else would come up." James recalled.

In 2016, James was driving and felt like he might swerve off the road. A week later, he was in the hospital. This was the beginning of his journey to a diagnosis of Lyme disease. James's disease took a lot from him, but the most difficult thing Lyme disease brought was the possibility he'd transmitted his disease to his daughter Yanissa. She had never been bitten by a tick but tested positive for the disease. "It's been a real challenge." James's voice broke. "I don't want to get too emotional, but it is hard. But we know God has a plan for us. The enemy tries to trip us up, but that's what's been so inspiring to me. I know God's plan for us must be so big the enemy's tried to take us down."

It wasn't a trail they had any control over, but they still had to climb, and they still are climbing. But both father and daughter have found purpose in the unmarked trail.

Yanissa strives to be an example to other teens to be kind to each other. "I think the biggest thing to understand is just because you look healthy on the outside does not mean you feel the same on the inside. I try to be compassionate to others." And James is impacting the world through the podcast, "Exercise Your Faith," he hosts with his friend and coworker, Dave McDonald.

An unmarked trail when climbing your mountain is not easy. It's taken me years to heal from the cruelty I experienced in high school, but there was beauty from the ashes. I learned empathy, compassion, and how important it is to make others feel that they matter. When you face an unmarked trail, remember God allowed it for a reason, so you will make it through. Don't do what I did by not sharing your doubts and burdens with other godly confidants who will pray for you and lift your spirits. This is biblical and what God wants you to do. If I had shared my heart with someone when I was in high school, then maybe I would have gained confidence and the self-worth to pursue opportunities sooner in my life. Once you cry out to God and take your focus off your problems, you will find purpose in the unmarked trail. Before you know it, you'll have conquered the trail and made it once again to your true course. But don't be surprised if it requires you to take a different path than you planned to get to your peak.

MOUNTAIN GUIDE TO THE NEXT PEAK:

1. Has anyone ever made you feel inferior for something you have no control over? What emotions did you feel?
2. What unmarked trails have you had to climb in your life?
3. What purpose did you find in them?
4. Did you ever talk to someone you trust about the pain and heartache you experienced? How did it help?
5. If you haven't released your burdens yet, take this time to write what you felt. Writing your thoughts, fears, and doubts is often the first step in the healing process.

_____

_____

_____

_____

_____

_____

_____

_____

_____

_____

_____

_____

_____

_____

_____

_____

_____

_____

A DIFFERENT PATH TO THE PEAK

Not all storms come to disrupt your life; some come to clear your path. —Unknown

Relief and freedom— I felt two emotions when I graduated from high school. Beaten and battered, I survived a severe storm while climbing my mountain, and now I witnessed a beautiful horizon—college.

I didn't realize at the time what college would hold for me. It would be a different path to the peak.

People wondered if college would be in my future because high school had been so difficult for me with my illness and numerous school absences. If I had shared those people's outlook on my life, I wouldn't have attempted college. But I never focused on my pain and the cannots. Instead, I focused on my joys and I cans. Yes, I missed many, many days of school because of sickness, but despite those difficult circumstances, I graduated on time with an excellent GPA and received multiple scholarships. I refused to allow my disease to define me. Instead, I defined my disease, and college would be another mountaintop victory.

I was determined to contribute to society and make a difference in this world. But I also knew I needed to choose a profession I could physically handle. I loved sign language, and I thought the hand gestures to form the signs were beautiful and graceful, so I decided to get a degree in deaf studies. It was a job I could do, and I would impact someone's life while doing it.

Accepted into Ohio University Southern, I could live at home, commute, and, since my sister also attended this university, we could carpool on some days. Everything fell into place. I loved the flexibility of college—I could choose my own classes, create my own schedule, and I enjoyed my sign language classes, as well as the professor who taught them. Everything was going so smoothly, and then uneven ground caused me to stumble when I discovered some signs I couldn't perform properly due to arthritis in my fingers. A setback like this would cause most people to take a step back, but not me. In fact, it was during this season of uncertainties God ignited a desire in my heart—to go to Asbury University, a school three hours away from home. I wasn't blind to the obstacles that made this dream seem impossible. My immune system was still fragile and I had a constant stream of infections. I had two to three doctor's appointments a month, and I took a monthly IV treatment. Going to Asbury didn't make sense and sounded like the perfect equation for disaster.

The desire grew stronger, and I knew it wasn't going away. I approached my parents one day and revealed to them what had been in my heart. The sudden halt in their activity told me I had shocked them. I wasn't the daughter they thought would go to Asbury, their alma mater. In their mind, my sister, who was healthy, would be the legacy student. My parents looked at each other and then at me. "Well ... that's an incredible dream you have, Sis," Mom said. "Why don't we all pray about it and see what doors God may open?"

"Okay," I agreed. I appreciated my parents' words. They didn't crush my dream by telling me it would never work. Instead, they were doing what they always did when, as a child, I tried to grab onto an unreachable dream—they let me try to reach it. But now, as a young adult, I could read their innermost thoughts in their eyes—*how would this ever work?*

I've heard it said when it rains, it pours, but with me, when it rains, there is also usually a tornado sighting.

Just as my dream of being a sign language interpreter was crashing around me, and the desire to go to Asbury University was beginning to bloom, my veins failed. Monthly IV sticks and multiple blood draws a month had taken their toll, and it took my nurses three to four tries to gain IV access for my treatment, sometimes more. My hematologist told me it was time to start thinking about getting a port, a medical device placed in a person's chest that allows direct access to a vein. But a CAT scan of my chest showed the veins and arteries in my chest were flowing in the opposite direction they should be.

"This is very unusual. There are always risks with port placements, mainly infections. But now your risks are much greater." Dr. Olshefski explained to me. "With the flow of your veins and arteries, deciding where to place a port is now difficult. And if it would ever become infected, it wouldn't be easy to remove. But you're the one being stuck multiple times, so this decision is up to you."

My tornado had touched down.

But my desire to go to Asbury became stronger. I never felt God cautioning this desire, and I continued to feel the gentle prodding to pursue my dream. At nineteen years old and battling a chronic illness, I lived in a safe little bubble with my parents and older sister. I needed to see to at what level I could function as an independent adult, balancing multiple tasks at once. I also longed for a college experience that would help heal the trauma I faced in high school. My aunt and her family had just moved to Wilmore, Kentucky, the small town where Asbury is located, so I had a support system if I needed one. I wanted to prove to everyone not only could I handle going away to school, but I could also graduate with my college degree while doing it. Most of all, I needed to prove it to myself. The thought of gaining my independence and reclaiming my sense of self-worth thrilled my soul.

My sister visited my aunt and her family, and while there, obtained a brochure explaining the college's mission and the degrees they had to offer. I looked at the pages with anticipation, and my heart leaped with joy when my eyes connected with creative writing. I loved to write, it was a career I could physically do, and I could make a difference in the world while doing it—God was making the path clear.

There are several types of climbing—rock climbing, alpine climbing, and mountaineering, just to name a few. There are different systems to show the difficulty of a mountain. Contributing expert Jay Parks of REI (a Seattle-based recreational equipment retailer) explains a popular one is the Yosemite Decimal System (YDS) and shares what that system entails. The mountain is assigned a *class* based on how technically difficult it is to climb. In class 1, the terrain is flat and can be walked. In class 2, the terrain is steeper, and the climber may need to use their hands to balance themselves. In class 3, the mountain incline is steeper than the previous class, and hands are now used. Some climbers may carry a rope if needed, and now, a small fall is possible. In class 4, most climbers carry ropes due to the incline's steepness, and longer falls are possible. In class 5, belayed roping is a must for safety, and climbing shouldn't be attempted by a beginner. A fall could lead to death in this class. Class 5 is divided into subcategories: easy, intermediate, hard, hard to difficult, and the final category, a class 6, can't be free climbed. The length of each climb is based on the difficulty of the path.[1]

The goal of every climber is reaching the summit, but the path to the top of the mountain may be different than they ever imagined. You plan to climb a class 1 mountain to get to your peak. Flat, simple to walk, easy as going from point A to point B. But the route changes, and God leads you to a path with the difficulty of a class 4 mountain where the terrain is steep, and a fall is possible.

That's what I was facing climbing life's mountains. My goal and desire were to get a college degree, and I wanted the degree to be deaf studies. When I discovered deaf studies would not be possible, it didn't deter my goal of obtaining my college degree. God was just leading me to a different path to get to the peak. Asbury University—check. Bachelor's in creative writing—check. Aunt as a support system if needed—check. I was climbing a class 3 mountain. The incline was steep, but now there was one obstacle blocking my view of the top—a clear way to maintain my medical care while attending a college five hours away from my team of specialists.

I was honored to host Jen Guiler on *Mountain Climbers* in November 2020. Like me, Jen knows the path you intend to take to the summit may not be the path that gets you there. Jen and her husband, Cody, got married, and like most couples, wanted to start a family. The young couple was unable to conceive after trying for a season. After much prayer, they felt God leading them on a different path. "After a year of trying, your relationship has taken a toll. We were ready to start a family. I don't need my children to be biologically related to me, and neither does Cody. We wanted kids, and we wanted them to be the children God wanted us to have. We knew our first baby would be through adoption, and then for subsequent kids, who knows? Who knows how God is going to work," Jen shared.

Jen and Cody decided to adopt domestically. Most adoption agencies are by state, so Jen reached out to a woman who lived in her area who had adopted a little girl, asking questions about adoption and what agency she went through. Jen and Cody began the agency's adoption process that included multiple conversations and a home study, which led to them getting approved. But the path was still not clear, and the couple faced the pain of the biological mother not following through with the adoption. "They have every right to make that decision, and that's the hardest part of adoption. Just knowing we are being called to support these people, but we may not get anything in return. It is hard, but it is so much of what Jesus asks us to do too. Once we took a step back from the pain and the hurt and the frustration, we could see that. For seven months, we were asked to love her, and we did that to the best of our abilities. And I think she'll always look back on that season of her life, and that's something." Jen said.

This painful journey was something Jen and Cody experienced again, and they had to process the emotions of pain, hurt, and frustration once more. But the couple's selfless love while longing to have a baby didn't go unnoticed by God, and they were matched with a beautiful baby boy they adopted and named Cameron. "Lots of people were at the hospital. We had social workers there, we had the expectant family, and they had a bunch of people there, we had a few people from our family—the day was very overwhelming. I remember the hospital gave us a room that night, and he got to stay in our room with us, and I remember just losing it after everybody left, and it was just Cody and me and Cam. It was just us, and I didn't have to put any guards up. It was just amazing. I'll never forget that moment." Jen smiled, recalling the day she met her son. Now God has doubly blessed Cody and Jen with a baby girl.

Just like God saw Jen and Cody's desire to have a baby, God also saw my desire to go away to school to get my college degree.

One day, I had a doctor's appointment with my immunologist. My mom and sister sat in the corner, my silent support system that day. As per routine, I told Dr. P how I had been doing between visits and if there had been any new developments, and this time I had a big new development. I remember telling him with a shrug, "I don't really want to get a port, but I probably will because I'm tired of getting stuck."

He looked at me with a smile. "You don't need to. There is a new treatment that was just approved for Children's. It's a subcutaneous version of your IVIg treatments, and it's given weekly instead of monthly. Being subcutaneous, it'll eliminate the need for multiple IV sticks, and since it's given weekly instead of monthly, the consistency will cut your infections down significantly."

At this point, I wanted to shout, "Sign me up!" Not as many needle sticks or infections? "I would love that!"

Again, Dr. P smiled. "Well, I haven't even told you the best part yet. Since your treatment is given subcutaneously instead of intravenously, you'll be giving it to yourself in the comfort of your own home. And since your infections will be so much better, you'll probably be able to go from monthly appointments with your specialists to every six months."

I looked over at my mom and sister. They knew, too. Mom smiled at me with tears in her eyes, and my sister's expression was a mix of excitement and sadness—her sister would be leaving her. "I get to go to Asbury."

Everyone's goal is to make it to their own personal peak. God has put a longing in all of us—we serve a victorious God who desires for his children to be victorious as well. But sometimes, we may have to take a different path to the peak than we planned. We may wonder why God led us to a different path—the other route was easy and sure. The Bible says in Proverbs 3:5 to trust in the Lord with all your heart and to lean not on your own understanding. This can be so difficult to do, but I promise, God wouldn't lead us to this path if he didn't have a specific purpose for us to climb it. Blessings, gifts, growth, healing, and revelations are waiting for us, and maybe, just maybe, unexpected doors and opportunities are on that trail too.

MOUNTAIN GUIDE TO THE NEXT PEAK:

1. What are some peaks you have wanted to reach in your life?
2. What path did you plan to take to reach the peak? Was it the path that led you to the top?
3. When God directed you to a different path to climb to your peak, what did you do?
4. What has this different path given you that you needed?
5. Has your path led you to your peak yet? How's the view?

_____

_____

_____

_____

_____

_____

_____

_____

_____

_____

_____

_____

_____

_____

_____

_____

_____

_____

AN UNEXPECTED TRAIL

Now unto him that is able to do exceeding abundantly above all that we ask or think, according to the power that worketh in us. —Ephesians 3:20

The appointment was about to wrap up.

"Oh, by the way, Whitney, I wanted to let you know I sent your case to the National Institutes of Health. There is a new disease called *DOCK8 immunodeficiency syndrome* an immunologist discovered there. You have similarities to the disease, and if the doctor thinks you fit the criteria of the protocol, you may get a phone call," Dr. P told me.

He had my interest. I had never heard of the National Institutes of Health or the NIH as most people call it, but I could sense its importance. All these years of living with an undiagnosed disease were normal to me, but at that moment, a little seed of hope bloomed in my heart, and I realized how much I needed the closure of a diagnosis. This opportunity came unexpectedly, and yet, I also knew at that moment, God was about to go exceedingly, abundantly above all I could ever ask or think.

A few months after my immunologist told me about that protocol possibility, I received a phone call from Helen Matthews, a nurse practitioner with immunologist Dr. Helen Su's research lab. "We are interested in your case and the potential it could fit into Dr. Su's DOCK8 protocol.

Before bringing you to the NIH for an in person visit, the next step is to get some research blood from you. Can the doctor who referred you, Dr. P, coordinate all of this with us?"

"Oh, yeah. I know he'd be more than happy to do that." My mind was going ninety miles an hour. It was surreal to me I was having this conversation.

"Okay, good. Once we get this blood and study it, we'll know if we can move forward with an in person visit. Now, I want to caution you, Whitney. There's a good chance we'll never figure out what's wrong with you. But you'll be invaluable research to us."

Even though I couldn't see her, I could hear the compassion in Helen's voice. It was obvious she had dealt with hopeful patients like me, who longed for answers. I understood why she cautioned me—Dr. Su and her team didn't want their patients to be crushed when they didn't receive breakthroughs. But I had this feeling within the depths of my soul I was about to embark on the most amazing journey I had ever been on.

Now, why wasn't my home immunologist's referral enough for me to be seen by Dr. Su and her team? The NIH is unique in how it operates. The NIH is a part of the US Department of Health and Human Services and is the nation's medical research agency.[1] The only way a person can become a patient or participate in a study at the NIH is by fitting the criteria listed in the protocol with the research physician's lab.

The NIH mailed the phlebotomy tubes to Dr. P at Nationwide Children's, I got the blood drawn, the vials of blood were mailed to Dr. Su's lab, and once again, it was a waiting game. But in the season of waiting, I was fulfilling my dream of getting my college degree at Asbury University. As a young woman who had insecurities and not much confidence, it took me a while to open up to others, but I bloomed in my junior year. A big reason for this was my roommate, Joy. She offered me the compassion and empathy I needed. We barely knew each other, and she still agreed to be my roommate. She was the Spiritual Life Advisor (SLA) to our hall our junior year, so she had seniority in choosing a room, and that room had a bathroom. My doctors urged me to seek a room with a bathroom to eliminate infections, and with that knowledge, she opened her room to me for our junior year of college.

Her mother had passed away from breast cancer when she was thirteen, so she had seen firsthand the toll illness could take on someone's body and how critical support and understanding are to someone battling a disease. She saw my invisible scars and encouraged me to see my own worth and step out of my comfort zone.

When I shared my story with those friends, they weren't skeptical of my authenticity or worry I might take some recognition from them as my high school classmates did. Instead, I was given acceptance, and they prayed God would grant me health. I gained the confidence to use my voice. The scars on my heart began to heal.

Looking back on my journey with the NIH and how it intertwined with my journey as a student at Asbury University, I can see clearly God knew what he was doing. He always does, right? He knew my broken pieces needed to be put back together so I could be ready for the purpose and calling he had for me that would come because of the NIH, and I needed to gain the boldness to speak and advocate for myself in ways I hadn't faced in my life. Asbury was the potter's wheel for God to take my pieces and put my vessel back together in a way so I could be used.

When it comes to climbing a mountain, REI explains knowing how to navigate the route chosen is critical to the climbers' success. Climbers should study guidebooks and websites of the mountain they are climbing. This helps the climber get a feel for what they will face when climbing that mountain—the form, terrain, and crevasses—giving them guidance on tackling the type of mountain they are attempting to climb. No matter the mountain, when the climbing team sets off on their journey, they must bring a map and compass to navigate the climb, and every climber should have the necessary knowledge to use both tools. A map and compass guide the climbers on the route they have planned and display what is ahead.[2] Preparing helps climbers know what to expect on the mountain, but it doesn't prevent the unexpected.

I have found this to be so true with life's mountains. As Christians, our map and guidebook is the Bible. By studying it, I gain the knowledge I need to climb life's mountains. I have salvation through God's son, Jesus Christ. I strive to know what God's teachings are and how to apply them to my life, so I can stand on God's promises and know God has a purpose for me. This is what I can expect. But it doesn't prevent the unexpected. In fact, the Bible shows us God often chooses to fulfill his promises in unexpected ways. Do you think Sarah thought she would have a baby at ninety? And how unlikely would it have seemed for hundreds of thousands of Israelites to escape the powerful Egyptian army through the parted Red Sea and on dry land, just because their leader stretched out his hand over the water? How many people doubted David could kill a nine-foot giant with a sling and a smooth stone? Even his brothers belittled him. And Mary, a young virgin, was the one God chose to carry his son, Jesus Christ. See? God's map does not always hold the expected, but it's peppered with beautiful, unexpected trails.

My journey to the NIH was one of those beautiful, unexpected trails. Just like God equipped David with a sling and a stone to slay Goliath, God used my dream of going to Asbury and the people I met there to equip me for what was ahead. By using God's map, I was learning who he created me to be.

Several months after the NIH studied my blood, I received the news I would be accepted into the DOCK8 protocol, and an inpatient visit would be planned. I would be climbing the unexpected trail.

Alex Baer, Jacob LeBrun, Gaven Traylor, and Sam Wiehle know the bountiful blessings and gifts that can come with an unexpected trail—the unlikely group of four launched The New Generation Quartet a few years ago. The young men were my guests on the fifteenth episode of *Mountain Climbers* (a milestone) and shared how God put their group together and orchestrated opportunities they could have never fathomed. Jacob said with a grin, "It's really neat how this all came together. I wanted to sing with Gaven, and we kind of got to talking and then wanted to add Alex in. Because Alex had been wanting to sing, but you know, he just kind of needed a little bit of a push to get there. We thought, *we'll do a trio*. And Sam was able to hear harmony well and had an excellent voice. Still does. So, we decided we'd add him in and form a quartet. And it all just kind of took off from there."

Jacob and Gaven were outgoing, so everyone knew they could sing—the surprise to everyone came with the shy Alex and Sam. As I told them in our interview, I didn't even know they could talk, let alone sing. So how did they get the push to step out of their comfort zone? "Actually, it was Jacob and my dad. 'Cause I always used to sing in the car, and he was like 'You need to start singing in church,' and I was like 'No, I'm way too nervous for that.' But then, when Jacob asked me to sing in the quartet, I was like, okay, this is my time, I got to do it." Alex said.

"I just remember, I always kind of wanted to sing, and I knew I could hear harmonies and stuff. I remember Jacob coming up to me and saying, 'Hey, if you join the group, then Alex will. Will you do it?' I was like, 'oh yeah ... sure,'" Sam said, imitating his hesitance when Jacob asked him, causing the other boys to chuckle. "From there, I remember that little push, and now here I am two years later. And I just don't know where I would be if I hadn't stepped out of my comfort zone."

The quartet made their debut at Rubyville Community Church's youth camp in front of their friends. Although nervous about how their friends would react to their singing, they sang for the Lord and the whole camp went crazy. "You know it's like everything else you do in life when you get support and encouragement, or someone says, 'Hey, you know you did a good job,' it really encourages you to keep going. To get better and to really get into it. The support we got after we sang at church camp and after we sang here (Rubyville Community Church) at our first church camp service that just motivated us to, you know, to better ourselves." Jacob spoke for the group.

They did keep going, and with God's map of an unexpected trail, two and half years later, opportunities and doors have opened for the quartet, including Sam and Gaven accepting the call to preach.

"We didn't mean for it to happen, but it was meant to be. So, when the stuff that's not in our hands starts to unfold, almost like it's laid out in front of you, that's probably when you just got be like okay this is what's supposed to happen," Gaven said with a smile. This is how God has done the unexpected with them, bringing the group together, and opening the doors for them.

That's the essence of God's map. There may be a lot of unexpected trails you would have never placed on your life's map. Still, I'm so thankful we serve a God who goes above anything we could ask or think—he did that with me when he opened the door for me to become a patient at the NIH and used my time at Asbury to prepare me for what was to come from my journey with the NIH. He did it with The New Generation Quartet, four random boys no one would put together, and he can do it for you. Don't dismiss that surprising trail—look for what you can learn as you climb it. See how God is healing you. Watch how he's using the unexpected trail as preparation for what's to come. The best aspect about unexpected trails? There's often a plateau where you can sit, rest, and bask in what God has done for you.

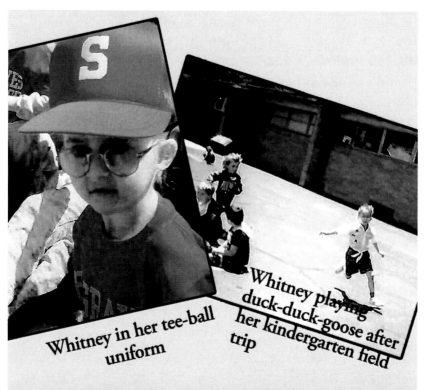

Whitney in her tee-ball uniform

Whitney playing duck-duck-goose after her kindergarten field trip

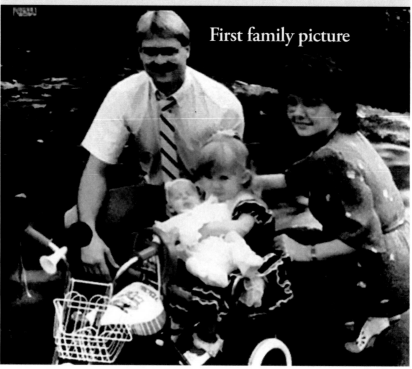

First family picture

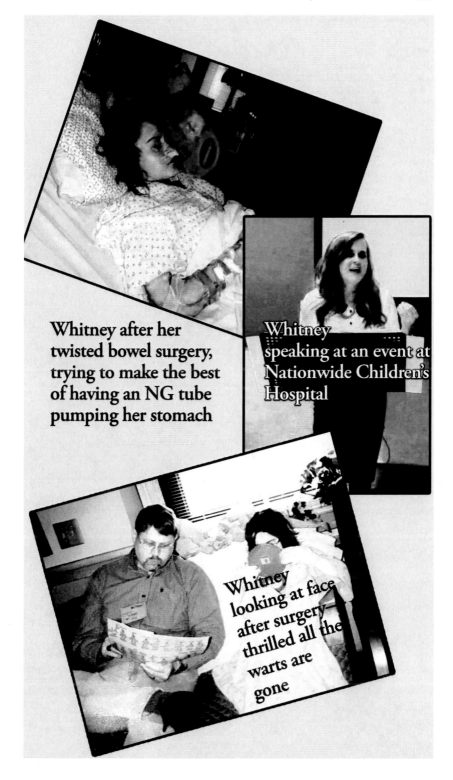

Whitney after her twisted bowel surgery, trying to make the best of having an NG tube pumping her stomach

Whitney speaking at an event at Nationwide Children's Hospital

Whitney looking at face after surgery thrilled all the warts are gone

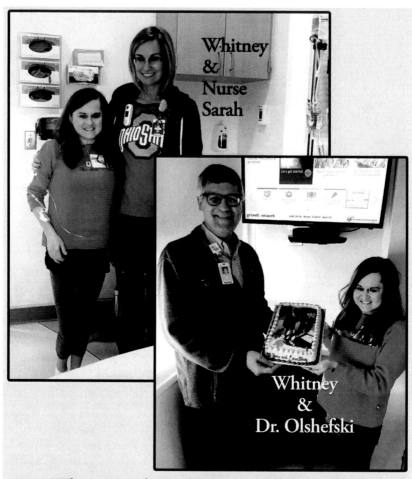

Whitney & Nurse Sarah

Whitney & Dr. Olshefski

Whitney with Dr. Higgins and Dr. Ardoin

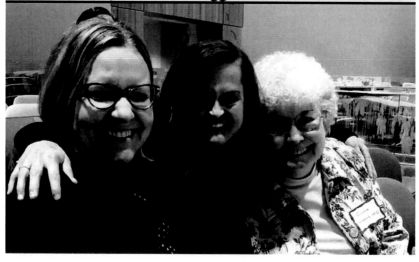

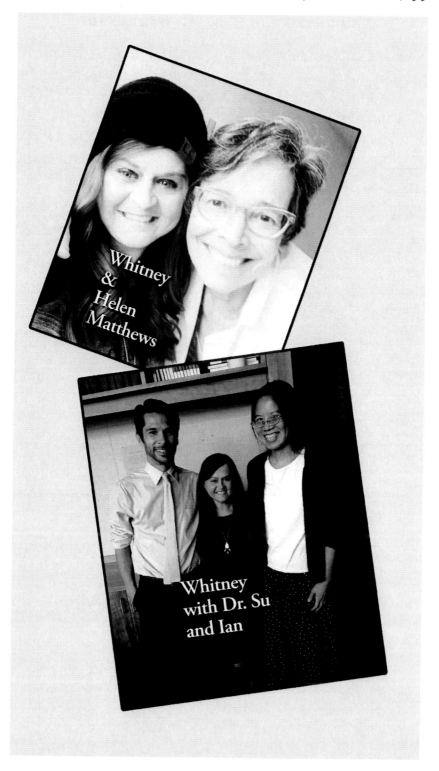

Whitney & Helen Matthews

Whitney with Dr. Su and Ian

MOUNTAIN GUIDE TO THE NEXT PEAK:

1. Have you ever climbed an unexpected trail? What was it?
2. Could you have ever fathomed the map God created for your life?
3. What did you learn? How did you heal? And how did God prepare you as you climbed your unexpected trail?

_____

_____

_____

_____

_____

_____

_____

_____

_____

_____

_____

_____

_____

_____

_____

_____

_____

_____

THE PLATEAU OF FRIENDSHIP

But they that wait upon the LORD shall renew their strength; they shall mount up with wings as eagles; they shall run, and not be weary, and they shall walk, and not faint. —Isaiah 40:31

"You hid behind your glasses," my mentor Lisa told me. Lisa was my mentor all the years I was at Asbury. After a rocky start, we formed a connection after Lisa was diagnosed with Crohn's disease. I helped her cope with the life changes that came with living with a chronic illness, and she helped me come out of my timid shell.

I pondered what she said. "You know, you're right, I did." My glasses had become a coping mechanism, helping me stay invisible. By wearing them, I didn't feel the need to put any effort into my appearance or do the little extra special touches that make a person feel good about themselves. But with my roommate, Joy's, constant encouragement and gentle pushes to put myself out there as well as Lisa challenging me to think more of myself than I did, I stepped out of my comfort zone in ways that showed healing had taken place in my heart—like wearing contacts and taking the time to apply makeup. Even as a new health development began—severe stomach pain and excessive weight loss, I still felt the burden of my insecurities melt away like winter transforming into spring.

In my junior year, I got to watch Joy fulfill her role as the SLA for our hall. I saw her pray and invest in the girls who lived with us. She managed meetings and events and had a special guest speaker share with the women from time to time. I loved the thought of investing in people in that way, I was ready to step into a similar leadership position, and I dreamed of this possibility for my senior year of college. But unfortunately, there was one issue—one of Joy's good friends was also interested in the position. So I pocketed the dream in my heart between God and me.

That summer, Joy and I went on a girls' trip to Pigeon Forge, Tennessee. I remember telling her how I thought I'd enjoy being an SLA.

"Oh, Whit!" she said with a smile. "I think you would make an amazing SLA."

"Thank you! If the position were open, I would love to go for it." I smiled and shrugged. I had accepted the door was closed.

"Oh, Jordy decided she didn't want it. As far as I know, the SLA position for our hall is still open."

The door had slowly cracked back open. "Really?"

"Yeah! You should totally apply." My roommate smiled at the growth she saw in me. The Whitney who approached her to see if she would consider being her roommate would not have had the confidence to seek out a role like this.

I mustered the boldness I needed, gathered my thoughts, and emailed the Spiritual Life Coordinator, (SLC). While waiting for an answer, I embarked on my first in-person visit to the NIH, with my parents accompanying me as my faithful support system.

When I think about the hotel we had to stay in the first couple of nights before moving to the NIH's on-campus housing, I always chuckle. I have never been in such a small space—there was barely a walking path, and with three adults in such a tiny area, it wasn't easy to move around in the room. However, this hotel managed to fit a chair in the corner of the room about a foot away from my bed. Propping my short legs on the bed, I got comfortable sitting in the chair using my computer to cruise through Facebook . After I signed off the social media website, I checked my email, and the email that was now in my inbox made my heart beat like a drum with excitement. The mail was from the SLC at Asbury, and his first sentence was, "Oh my goodness, this is an answer to prayer! The position is yours!" I was on cloud nine the rest of the evening, and it gave me hope that led into what would be an exhausting and long week.

I was in awe when I stepped inside the NIH campus that sits on 300 acres and boasts more than seventy-five buildings—it looked like a little city.[1] I spent my week at the Clinical Center, where clinical research participants are seen. I've never walked so much or seen as many specialists in one day, let alone the whole week.

If my team thought I needed to see a doctor, they called for an appointment to see the specialist the same day.

I was appreciative when I discovered Dr. Su, Helen Matthews, and the rest of Dr. Su's team saw me as a human and not a petri dish to decipher. They didn't just want to know about my medical history. They wanted to know what made me, me. In fact, every single researcher and specialist I saw during that week viewed me as a person first and a patient second. This was so refreshing. I was more open and flexible to do what was asked of me because I knew they cared, and they put my best above a scientific find.

By the end of my visit, I knew I didn't have DOCK8, but Dr. Su wanted to keep me as a patient and continue researching my undiagnosed illness. That was the good news. The bad news was they discovered the stomach pain I had and the weight I was losing was due to a twisted bowel. Worse, it had to be surgically repaired.

"I can't have surgery right away. I just accepted a leadership position at my college. I'm not giving it up. Can

I wait and have my surgery during Christmas break? I can combine my last two weeks of college for the semester, so I can have an extra week to recover during my break." I know my doctor could see my heart in my eyes as I begged her to approve of the plan.

"I think that'll be okay, but you need to lay out this plan with your home surgeon and make sure he signs off on it as well. But I wouldn't wait any longer than that," Dr. Su cautioned.

I'm so thankful I advocated for my wishes because otherwise, I would have missed out on something special—the plateau of friendship. I arrived on campus early because I had to attend SLA training. I walked into the building and looked for a friendly person, someone I could connect with. I saw a girl sitting on a couch by herself, so I sat beside her and introduced myself.

"Hi, I'm Whitney."

"Hi! I'm Kelli."

"It's nice to meet you. So what dorm are you an SLA for?"

"Aldersgate," she replied referring to apartments for upperclassmen.

"Oh, me too!" I said with excitement. "Well, for the Sarah Johnson building. This is great. We'll have meetings together then."

"Aww, yes, this is perfect!"

This was the beginning of a unique and special friendship. Kelli and I clicked so quickly, and I'll never forget the day during SLA training our friendship was solidified as sisters of the heart. Kelli and I decided to have lunch in her apartment instead of going to the cafeteria. I asked her how old she was.

"I'm 21."

"I'm 23. I actually just had a birthday."

"Me too!" Kelli said.

"Really? My birthday is in August."

Kelli gasped. "So is mine."

Okay, surely our birthdays aren't on the same day. What are the odds? "My birthday is August 1st."

Kelli's eyes grew round, and her mouth dropped. "My birthday is on August 1st too! Oh, my goodness, this is such a gift from Jesus!"

She was right—but what I didn't count on was how many gifts Jesus would give me during that week of SLA training.

Along with Kelli, I met with Aldersgate's SLA staff every other week, and we were considered the upperclassman housing on campus. The SLC who gave me the position was replaced by my friend Annie. Annie and I were both majoring in creative writing and had already begun a friendship. Our SLA group consisted of six women and two men who God beautifully and wonderfully knitted together in friendship and leadership.

I'd always dreamed of being a part of such a tight-knit group of friends. I loved having two guy friends who became my brothers and protectors and dubbed me "Li'l Whit," which became my name of endearment in the group. What made our group so special is how close we became despite being juniors and seniors. The Aldersgate SLA staff hadn't formed into such a close group in the past because, being upperclassmen, most students had already established friendship groups or had significant others they spent most of their time with. It became known on campus how close we were, and our SLA program director noted our bond was unusual, calling us a posse. I think God knew how much my heart needed these friendships for my climb.

When it comes to climbing a mountain, *wikiHow* stresses one of the most important climbing codes of ethics is don't climb alone. Now you may be thinking—wait, hasn't she already touched on this? You're right. I have. But this is a point stressed in the world of mountain climbing, so I'm repeating it. This time applying it to friendship, not professionally. Every person brings something to a climb—different gifts and skills they excel at. One climber may be sharper one day than the other. The next day, another climber might have a perspective needed for that stage in the climb.[2] And again, *Sportrock* explains the importance for the climber to have a belayer to manage the rope from the bottom of the mountain.[3] It doesn't matter how many classes a climber has taken, how many clubs they are a part of, or how much research or guidebooks they have read. The fact remains climbing with others is vital to success and safety.[2]

Likewise, this mountain climbing application bears repeating for life's mountains—don't climb your mountain alone. It might be your personal mountain to face, but the key to success and safety is to surround yourself with friends who can pray for you and encourage you to keep climbing even when the incline gets steep. You can confide in them about the burden you're carrying because they will help you carry it—a *burden carrier* belayer.

One of my favorite Bible stories is when the Israelites fought the Amalekites. The key to the Israelites' victory was Moses raising his hands. Eventually, Moses became tired and was losing the strength to continue holding his hands up. So his brother, Aaron, and a man named Hur provided Moses a stone to sit on, and then they held his arms in the air, so the Israelite Army would win the battle.

This is what you need—arm holders—people who will hold your arms, support you, and let you lean against them when you're losing the strength to climb. The wonderfully deep foundation about these friendships is those people won't just be there with you in difficult times. Instead, they will be there to celebrate with you when you reach your summit.

Last March, I had the honor of launching a spin-off of *Mountain Climbers*—*Mountain Climbers: Youth Edition*. My first guests were the Rubyville Community Church Youth officers, Sam, Jacob, Hannah, and Mckenna. I loved the vision of friendship and community they wanted to incorporate within the group.

"There are three main parts we're focusing on. Growth would be the first one. Over the last year or so, we've experienced a lot of growth in our youth, and we want to continue to see it grow. Also, unity—this year, there's a big gap between the older kids and the younger kids. We want to see them unite and just grow stronger in the Lord, and the closer they grow with each other, the closer they will get to God. So we're working on creative ways to kind of get them to talk to each other and unite," Hannah Arthur, who acted as the youth secretary and is presently the youth president spoke for the officers.

This interview took place a month before the COVID pandemic induced a nationwide lockdown. What made me so proud of these four youth officers is the pandemic didn't keep them from what they set out to do when elected. They connected with the other teens in the youth program through email, text messages, and Zoom meetings, offering their support, encouragement, and confirmation those kids had arm holders to help them climb the mountain they were facing.

After the week of training, I came to see I had a whole army of arm holders. In the middle of the week, more and more students trickled back on campus to gear up for the new semester. I had a lunch break in between training, so I made my way to the cafeteria. I put my stuff at a table, then went to get some food. I checked out what the different buffets had, and I was stopped by a friend who squealed, "Hey, Whitney!" and gave me a big hug. We talked about our summers and made plans to have a lunch date. After we were done chatting, I got some food from the buffet, walked it back to my table, and proceeded to go back to another buffet. Once again, I was "hug tackled" by another friend who'd just arrived on campus. We chatted for a few minutes, made plans to hang out, and I continued my quest to find food. And lo and behold, I ran into another friend, and then another, and then another.

I finally walked back to my table with my lunch. I didn't know if I would have time to eat before the next training, but my heart soared with joy at the plateau of friendship I basked in. At that moment, the Lord whispered an epiphany to the depths of my soul. *You see, Whitney, you didn't have this in high school, but if you had, what you have now wouldn't mean as much.* He was right. The friendship, community, and comradery I now had were like a soothing balm to my heart. My favorite verse immediately came to mind—*But they that wait upon the LORD shall renew their strength; they shall mount up with wings as eagles; they shall run, and not be weary, and they shall walk, and not faint. —Isaiah 40:31.*

I had waited and did not grow weary in due season, and now I had a renewed strength that came from my arm holders—my plateau of friendship. When God gives you those gifts and blessings your heart longed for, for so long, there's only one enterprise to initiate. You shout it from the mountaintop.

MOUNTAIN GUIDE TO THE NEXT PEAK:

1. Why is it so important to not climb your mountains alone?
2. What's an arm holder mean to you?
3. How wonderful God doesn't make us climb our mountains alone. Take a moment and thank God for the friends who encourage you, pray for you, and hold your arms up—your plateau of friendship.

_____

_____

_____

_____

_____

_____

_____

_____

_____

_____

_____

_____

_____

_____

_____

_____

_____

_____

_____

SHOUT IT FROM THE MOUNTAINTOP

God uses our trials to build our faith, draw us closer
to Him, and give us a testimony of His faithfulness for
others to see. —Dr. Michelle Bengston

On my first night at Asbury, I lay in my bunk after an
intense day of orientation, and a dream took root—I wanted
to share my story in chapel. Ironically, my timidity did
not deter me. I could envision myself on stage telling the
student body what I had been through, but how God was
faithful every step of the way. Perhaps God saw the woman
I would grow into? Whatever the reason, this dream was
born, and just as I did with my desire to be an SLA, I tucked
it in the depths of my heart where God could see it but
never told anyone.

I was so excited for my first meeting with the girls in
my hall as their SLA. Watching Joy the year before, I got
tons of ideas. In her first meeting, she and the Resident
Advisor (RA) shared their testimonies. I wanted to do this
as well, so the women we were ministering to in my hall
could relate to me and the RA.

I made an ice cream sundae dessert for the event, got
my room ready, stepped out of my room, and shouted
Koinonia, the word for all SLA small group gatherings, a
Greek word meaning "fellowship," at the top of my lungs.
I was nervous, as I always was when I shared my story, but

I was ready. The RA shared her testimony first, and then, I told my story. The women were so receptive, and what I didn't know at that time, a seed was planted in one girl's heart.

A couple of months later, some classmates in my fiction writing class decided to attend a literary reading together. Going to three local author readings that semester was a part of our class's curriculum. That same woman who attended the first *Koinonia* I held was also in my writing class.

"Hey, Whitney, are you going to the reading tonight?" she asked as we were leaving class.

"Yeah, I'm going. Are you?"

She smiled. "Yes, I am. I need to talk to you about something tonight before or after the reading."

"Okay." I smiled back. But my insides crashed like waves at high tide. My analytical, overthinking everything, nature kicked in. I knew this woman, and we had a history. I met her on the first day of orientation when we were divided into groups. We were both transfer students and were in the same orientation group. We didn't have the same circle but were friends and had bonded over our diminutive statures.

What does she want to talk to me about? Did I do something? Is she talking to me for someone else? To this day, confrontation of any sort makes me go weak in the knees, and that's what I thought I was about to face.

I rode to the reading with my friend Annie. It was pouring the rain that night, which added to my trepidation of doom. We arrived and were seated with about five minutes to spare. My friend who wanted to speak with me sat about two seats away. She looked at the writing friend who was sitting next to me. "Do you care to switch me seats really quick so I can talk to Whitney?" They switched, and she sat beside me. *Here we go...*

"So I'm the student chair on the committee that chooses chapel speakers. I help select student chapel speakers.

After you shared your story, I just thought you would be an amazing student speaker. So, I want to know, would you be willing to share your testimony in chapel?"

My reaction? I bawled. The surprise, honor, and answer to prayer wrecked me.

"Ahhh," she patted my shoulder. "Are you okay?"

"Yes," I said through sobs. "I'm just so happy. This is a dream come true for me."

She gave me a side hug. "I'm glad you're happy about this. You'll be speaking on November 7. So two weeks from today."

It was an exciting but intense two weeks of preparing what I was going to say. During student chapel, two students spoke and had twelve minutes each to share what was in their hearts. In those twelve minutes, I wanted to tell my story in a relatable way, which would speak to and encourage the student body. In some ways, the two weeks moved so slowly, and in other ways, the time flew by. But the day did arrive, and even though I was nervous, I was ready.

My parents, sister, grandparents, aunt, uncle, and cousins were there to support me. The chapel service began, the worship team sang, and then, my roommate Joy introduced me to the twelve hundred students in attendance. I walked to the free-standing microphone and adjusted it. And it went limp. I adjusted it once more, and again it fell, pointing to the ground as if all the traction had left the mechanism. The auditorium abrupted in awkward laughter. Sheer panic filled my soul. *This is so embarrassing ... I only have twelve minutes, and this is eating into my time!*

Out of the corner of my eye, I saw the worship leader head to the stage to assist me. I raised the microphone in one more attempt. It did a 360° flip and stopped where I needed it. Relief flooded my soul. I smiled at the audience and flashed a thumbs-up as they laughed and clapped in support. I have no doubt God's hand was holding the microphone, and now, the ice was broken, and I had everybody's attention. For the next twelve minutes, I shouted from the mountaintop about God's faithfulness. I spoke about my disease and the uncertain seasons it brought. I told of the beautiful opportunities at Asbury, which led to a plateau of friendship I always longed to have. I told them when I didn't have the strength to go to where God was, he came to me. I also told them what God had done for me, he would do for them if they would trust in him.

As I ended my testimony, relief and peace filled my soul. I had given my peers the message God wanted them to hear. Countless students and faculty passed by after chapel was over to tell me I did a good job and how much they needed to hear what I said. I beamed from ear to ear, not knowing the irony of the words I spoke, "When I didn't have the strength to go to where God was, he came to me" would take on a whole new meaning in just a month.

The friendships I had and being recognized as a leader on campus lifted my spirit in incredible ways. But it didn't hide the signs. I was so sick. I needed the semester to heal my heart and the feelings of insecurity and inferiority I had but living with a twisted small intestine took a toll on my body. The weight continued to fall off at an alarming rate, and my appearance took on a look of skin and bones. My hair was constantly shedding, becoming thin like I was, as I brushed out tangles and knots daily. One of the worse developments was it became difficult to know what to eat and drink. Foods I normally loved caused my stomach to cramp, and I would double over in pain.

But I didn't quit. Instead, I strove to do my best in all areas of my life—investing in the women on my hall as their SLA, being an intentional friend, and getting good grades in all my classes. Combining the week of final projects and finals week was brutal, and they stretched me thin, but I didn't just finish, I finished well. I was proud of what I accomplished in such dire circumstances.

The day my parents and sister came to pick me up for my surgery, Joy and I ate brunch in the cafeteria. As we walked out, she slung her arm around my neck. "Well, this is your last meal in the cafeteria this semester."

"Yeah ... if I come back."

"Whitney! Don't say that," she said. Her tone and wide eyes displayed her chagrin.

I smiled and shrugged. I didn't know how to respond, and I just had a sense of foreshadowing I was about to be in the fight of my life. Further confirmation of what I felt in my spirit happened that day. My parents, sister, and I had dinner with my aunt and cousin before we got on the road to head for home. I hugged my cousin and aunt bye, and I started crying. "Ahh, why are you crying?" my cousin asked in compassion. She never saw me face medical obstacles with tears or dread, only determination and steel. My aunt saw my tears. "She's never faced anything like this kind of surgery, and she's nervous."

She was right. This surgery was unlike any I had ever faced. With a colonoscopy and an endoscopy included in the surgery, I would be unable to eat for a couple of days before. When I awoke from the surgery, an NG tube would be in my nose to pump my stomach until it produced bowel sounds, a sign my stomach had healed from the surgery. Until those sounds were heard through a stethoscope, I was not permitted to eat—and no one knew when that would happen. A month prior, I was shouting on the rooftop of God's faithfulness and his good gifts. Now I was facing an uncertain mountain. A mountain that I felt would lead to a season where my life would hang in the balance.

Jeff Bonaldi wrote in "14 Fast Facts about Mount Everest," that Mount Everest, at 29. 029 feet. is one of the most dangerous mountains to climb, and it takes days to conquer. Remarkably, over four thousand people have climbed Mount Everest.[1] Sadly, Hillary Bruek with *Business Insider* reports that over three hundred people have succumbed to the mountain.² Ironically, Grayson Schaffer's *Washington Post* article tells of five myths of Mount Everest, and one is Mount Everest is not a technically difficult mountain to climb. What makes the famous mountain deadly is the cold winter environment—avalanches, ice collapses, high-altitude pulmonary and cerebral edema, falls, dysentery, stroke, and hypothermia.³ In another *Washington Post* piece, Sarah Kaplan points to the dangers of the Khumbu Icefall located at the head of the Khumbu Glacier. She explains the glacial wonder is one of the most dangerous sections of Mount Everest because the Khumbu Icefall shifts and reshapes itself due to its enormity. Crevasses seem to form, and monstrous ice towers, known as seracs, have the reputation of collapsing. The danger of the Khumbu Icefall is so notorious mountain climbers have given it the aliases of the Popcorn Field and Ballroom of Death.⁴

Some mountains we face in life are small. The climb was hard, but it was quick. It took no time to make it to the top, God orchestrated the details and solutions, and just as fast as it formed, the mountain was conquered. But some mountains we face are Mount Everest. The climb is difficult and will take an unsurmountable time to climb because of how monstrous it is. The hazards you'll experience will make the climb dangerous, especially when some of those experiences are like a Khumbu Icefall wreaking havoc.

I didn't know what the outcome of my climb would be. I made it through my surgery beautifully. The NG tube ranked in the top five medical treatments I hated, but I tolerated it. The most difficult aspect of the surgery was not being able to eat until my small bowel had healed. If it were taken out too soon, then any food I consumed would not stay in my stomach but regurgitate in the form of black vomit. If that happened, the NG tube would have to be re-inserted. My first NG tube had been placed after I had been put to sleep for my surgery. I didn't have to be told that an NG tube placement was painful, and it was a blessing I was asleep when it was put in. I was dreading the tube being removed while awake, but the thought of it having to be put in terrified me. Yes, it was hard not to be able to eat, but I'd take a gurgling stomach crying out for food over black vomit and an NG tube being forced through my nose and into my throat until it reached my stomach.

My surgeon took pity on me and allowed me to have a popsicle every four hours. It was fascinating to eat a popsicle and, thirty minutes later, watch the NG tube pump it out of my stomach. Finally, after eight days of not eating, my small intestine worked again, and I was allowed to eat. The next day I was discharged, and I went home. My hemoglobin was a little lower than normal due to the trauma of surgery, but normal for what my body had experienced. I was exhausted, and the scale said I weighed a whopping seventy-five pounds, but I was happy to be home and start the road to gaining my health back.

Over the years, I have found victory isn't always about making it to the top of the mountain, but it's how you handled the climb. Did you complain about the hardships you were facing while climbing the mountain, or did you get to the point where you could say, "This is hard, but you know what … God's got this." Did you focus on the mountain's size, or did you shift your focus to find purpose during the climb? Did you allow the dangers of the climb to immobilize you with fear? Or did you climb despite the fear, knowing when you placed your faith and trust in God, he would give you the strength to climb?

One *Mountain Climbers: Youth Edition* guest who comes to mind when I think of these victorious qualities is Jocelyn Cooper. What makes the way she's faced her Mount Everest so admirable is she was only sixteen years old when she found her purpose in the midst of her climb. With Jocelyn's parents both being drug addicts, she fended for herself at a young age. Her father left home when she was a little girl, and while her mother didn't bring drugs into the home, she often was absent to quiet the beast of addiction. Eventually, Jocelyn's home life took a toll on her, and she acted out—drinking, hanging out with the wrong crowd, and skipping school. "My grades were all 'F's,' and even when I did go to school, I was on in-school suspension or arguing with teachers. Even during all of that, I still went to church. I don't know what part of me was like, getting into trouble is okay, but I still went to church," Jocelyn shared.

It was obvious God had a unique and special purpose for Jocelyn. Soon, Jocelyn's principal noticed her behavior and the fact there was a lack of parental supervision in Jocelyn's life. Her principal reached out to her aunt and mother's sister, Sonia. "My principal ended up contacting Sonia and telling her I just wasn't safe where I was, and about me not going to school and getting into trouble. And on April 6, 2017, I moved in with Sonia and Chris. I was thirteen."

After Jocelyn's dad passed away, God put the vision and calling on Jocelyn's heart for what she was born to do. "I found, after my dad passed away, that he'd gotten saved. A lot changed after that especially, and even though it was hard, I wanted to help other people who were going through the same thing," Jocelyn said with a smile. "And let them know they don't need to lose faith and hope. Even with bad things, a lot of good things can come."

With the help of Sonia and many others, Jocelyn launched Directly Affected, a community peer support program led by teens to help teens who have a loved one in their life who is battling addiction. Directly Affected offers these teens a safe place to share their burdens of being affected by the drug epidemic and their loved one's choices. To teens facing a similar mountain, Jocelyn has a special message. "Never lose faith. Always have faith. And always have hope. And don't stop praying. Just pray, pray, pray. And God will help you come out of any situation you are in. He has a plan for every single one of you, and you just need to try to stay on it no matter what's happening in your life. And keep climbing." Jocelyn smiled and threw her hand in the air with emphasis.

Although Jocelyn faced a different mountain than me, they were both Mount Everest type mountains in our lives. And we both tackled our mountains in the same way— by choosing to find purpose during the climb. But my foreboding premonition hadn't yet manifested. A storm was brewing on my Mount Everest. I was about to see that continuing to climb and finding purpose isn't always enough to protect you from the dangers of life's Mount Everest. Sometimes it takes the supernatural—angel first aid.

MOUNTAIN GUIDE TO THE NEXT PEAK:

1. Think of the blessings God's given you. What miracles and gifts from God would you shout from the mountaintop?
2. Have you ever faced a Mount Everest in life? How did it make you feel?
3. How did you handle your climb in a victorious way?

_____

_____

_____

_____

_____

_____

_____

_____

_____

_____

_____

_____

_____

_____

_____

_____

_____

_____

ANGEL FIRST AID

Be not forgetful to entertain strangers: for thereby some
have entertained angels unawares. —Hebrews 13:2

The vomiting, crippling fatigue, lack of color in my
cheeks, and fading tint of red in my gums and eyelids—all
pointed to one horrifying possibility—a hemolytic crisis.
My dad didn't even have time to change out of his work
clothes before we headed back to Nationwide Children's
a little over twenty-four hours after being discharged
from my surgery. The on-call hematologist my mom spoke
with notified the ER we were coming, but the ER was still
slammed that night. After I was triaged, the nurse put my
parents and me in a private room adjacent to the ER waiting
room to wait for a room. I slumped over in my wheelchair,
praying I would be called to the back soon.

"Hey, honey," my mom began. "While we're sitting here,
I want to tell you something."

"What?" *Something to take my mind off how miserable
this is?*

"Well, the Lord told me he is going to heal you in the fall."

"He did?"

Mom smiled. "Yes, he did. I wasn't sure if I heard
correctly at first, but God kept putting it on my heart. I
told your dad. But I haven't found a good time to tell you
since your semester has been so crazy."

"When? How?" I never questioned my mom's words. My faith told me my mom heard God. I thought about what life could be like with a healthy body. I imagined what I could do without a compromised immune system.

"I don't know that. All I know is, it's going to happen."

"Well, that's so amazing." My heart soared at the possibilities on the horizon.

Around midnight, I settled into a room in the ER. After multiple sticks, an IV was placed—a sure sign I was dehydrated. Then, two hematology interns entered my room, laid out their plan, and had some surprising news to deliver.

"So your hemoglobin is actually 8.4."

"Really? It's that high?" Mom's high-pitched voice mirrored the confusion the three of us felt. My symptoms suggested a much lower hemoglobin.

While an 8.4 wasn't the greatest level, it wasn't at a level yet where I would need a blood transfusion. Because I'd received several blood transfusions over the years, I had inherited the antibodies of those donors. When the blood bank matched my blood, they couldn't look only at my O positive blood type. Instead, they had to match all the antibodies present in my blood as well. It became more difficult to match my blood with each blood transfusion, and it took hours for the blood bank to find the best possible match.

"Yeah, so that's the good news." The intern half-smiled. Proof there was indeed bad news. "We're going to admit her and monitor her. We'll give her fluids and probably go ahead and give her Rituxan treatment even though she's not due for it yet." The intern did her best to connect with all three of us. "The bad news is that the hematology floor is full." Her tone was low, and her features drawn. "We won't be able to get you in there right now." She knew she'd delivered a blow.

"Okay." My attitude to deal with what was handed to me with level-headed calm took hold and steeled me for whatever might come—with the dread I also felt taking its place right behind it.

"Just curious, do you know what floor she will go to until she can go to hematology?" My dad asked.

The intern nodded her head. "Yeah, she'll go back to the surgery floor. But we won't give her Rituxan until she is on the hematology unit."

The floor I was on forty-eight hours ago—a staff who took good care of me post-surgery but was not trained to look for the signs of a dangerously low hemoglobin. Mom, Dad, and I looked at each other with wide eyes and pursed lips. This was not good.

That Tuesday was what nightmares are made of. My parents watched me deteriorate before their eyes. My color went from pale to yellow to white. I couldn't go to the bathroom without my dad carrying me and then anchoring me, so I didn't fall off the commode. My urine went from a healthy yellow to a disturbing shade of dark brown. Every time I stood before going to relieve myself, a knife sliced through my head. I went from being able to carry conversations with my parents to only having the strength to nod or shake my head to communicate.

My parents were at a loss on what to do. The bag of fluids was not making a difference, and the surgical staff's only course of action was to take vitals more frequently. We all breathed a sigh of relief when my hematologist, Dr. Olshefski, walked through the door. His expression became ashen, and the worry lines on his face became prominent. He was used to a patient with quick comebacks and snarky one-liners—not one who was only capable of staring.

He stood by my bed and looked at me as he whispered to my parents. "I'm told by the on-call hematologist she will be moved tonight to the hematology floor. She'll be given her Rituxan, but because her hemoglobin was 8.4 early this morning, they don't plan on drawing labs again until tomorrow morning. But when you get to the floor tonight, you need to insist they do it tonight. It's imperative they do not wait."

My parents were crushed. "Okay." They agreed—ready to do battle for their daughter's life.

"And if she makes it ... we may need to talk about a bone marrow transplant."

His message was subtle, but my dad caught it. "Did you hear what he said?" he asked my mom after Dr. Olshefski left my room. "He said 'if she makes it.' He doesn't think she's going to make it."

One of the most well-known mountain-climbing tragedies happened on Mount Everest in May of 1996, commonly known as the "Everest Disaster." The experience was traumatic, and many books were written about the calamity, including *Into Thin Air* by journalist Jon Krakauer, which became a bestseller. The History Channel's website reported on May 10th, four different expeditions had the same goal—make it to the top. Out of nowhere, a devastating blizzard struck. With many climbers at high altitudes, the feeling of euphoria evaporated with the dire circumstances. Even the more experienced mountaineers struggled to climb due to the severity of the winter storm. Eight climbers died that day, setting a record as the largest number of lives lost on Mount Everest to happen in a single day.[1]

Sometimes in life, not only do mountains the size of Mount Everest loom, but destructive storms can also appear while you're climbing that could threaten your life. I was facing a storm on Mount Everest.

There's a person I would love to have on *Mountains Climbers*, and if she hadn't lived centuries before me, I would have. I love her story, and to me, she's the essence of who a mountain climber is—the woman with an issue of blood. When it comes to people in the Bible, I've always felt a connection with her. We both know what it's like to live with unusual illnesses affecting our blood. She tried everything. No doctor could cure her and gave her no hope of healing. She faced a storm on Mount Everest as well. But she had faith. I can picture as the doctor left one final time, telling her he had done all he could do—she fell onto the ground in tears. Then, a determination and sense of righteous indignation filled her spirit. I can see her as she rose, clenched her fists, and mustered the last bit of strength to go to Jesus, uttering the words, "If I may touch but his clothes, I shall be whole." She was made whole just by touching the hem of his garment.

I didn't have the strength to go to Jesus, but just like the woman with the issue of blood, even during my storm, I had faith.

When I was moved to the hematology floor, my parents did what Dr. Olshefski told them to, and a plan was quickly put into place.

"Hey, Whitney." My nurse entered my dark room—no lights and hushed voices, I could not be over-stimulated. "We need to get you up and weigh you so we can get your Rituxan ordered."

"She just said she had to go to the bathroom." Mom told him.

"Okay, well, why don't we get both of those things over with."

The nurse began helping me. "My head hurts so bad." I panted.

"Okay, we'll take it slow."

It was no use. The movement and stimulation were too much. My stomach heaved, and the force of the convulsion caused my bladder to release. Terror filled my heart as I took in the coal-black substance all over the bed. *Oh no, they are going to put an NG tube in my nose again!* But humiliation took over as I realized I was soaked in my own vomit and urine.

"It's okay. You're okay," The nurse assured me. "I want you to lay back down. Dad, why don't you stand beside her head while Mom and I clean her up."

My dad bent beside me and stroked my forehead. Hot tears filled my eyes and spilled onto my cheeks. "This is so embarrassing," I whispered.

"You can't help this. So, don't worry about it." Dad whispered back.

"So, Whitney, you're in college, right?" The nurse seemed to sense my mortification.

"Yeah."

"What are you studying?"

"Creative writing."

"Oh, really? That's awesome. Tell me about some of the stuff you have written."

I smiled. I had just turned in a portfolio for my fiction writing class. My characters were fresh on my mind. "Well, I wrote a story called 'The Discovery.' It's about an archeologist professor named Dr. Harold Moots, who works at Oxford—"

My clarity of mind, lucidity, and ability to form coherent thoughts disappeared at that moment, and I rambled like a mad person. My mom later told me it was as if all my stories, characters, and plots got jumbled and twisted—nothing I said made sense. I went in and out of consciousness, and in the rare moments my eyes were opened, I was locked within my body, incapable of moving, speaking, or acknowledging my surroundings. My blood pressure dropped to sixty over thirty, making a heart attack a scary reality.

It took many attempts for the nurses to get any blood from my veins. When they did get the smallest drop, they would run it to the lab, but by the time they got it to the lab, the blood had already clotted. Finally, they raised my bed as high as it would go, dangled my arm over the bed, and squeezed my arm from my armpit to the tip of my finger to retrieve one drop of blood, which was rushed to the lab.

"Why don't you go get a shower while we're waiting for the results, and I'll stay with her." My dad told my mom.

Dad pleaded with me to talk to him. "C'mon Whitney, it's Dad. Please talk to me. 'Jesus loves me, this I know, for the Bible tells me so.'" At a loss for what to do, he sang the first song that came to mind. I stared at him. I could hear him. I knew he was begging me to speak, to reassure him I was okay, but my body wouldn't let me form the words. Back into the blackness I went.

Thirty minutes later, five doctors entered my room with devastating news. Dad knocked on the bathroom door. "Cathy, hurry and get back to Whitney's room now. Her hemoglobin is 3.4. They want to take her to the ICU."

Five minutes later, Mom rushed into my room. "Whitney's hemoglobin is 3.4?" She demanded.

Before the other doctors could answer, the hematologist interns I saw in the ER came running in out of breath. "We just came from the lab." One the interns said between breaths. "It's actually 2.8."

"What are we going to do about blood? Her hemoglobin was 8.4 Monday night. She's not transfused at 8.4. It takes hours to get blood for her. She doesn't have hours." Mom summoned her last strand of calmness.

The other hematology intern spoke. "We expected the 8.4 on Monday could be a false high due to dehydration. So we ordered blood that night. It's here. We don't have to wait on it."

"Thank you." My mom said through tears.

"Okay, let's get some oxygen on her." The ICU attending physician placed the tubes in my nose.

My eyes opened in shock as the tube in my nose gave my body the oxygen it lacked. Then, I noticed all the doctors in my tiny hospital room.

My mother saw the terror in my eyes and that I was ready to bolt from the bed. She leaned close and caressed my brow. "Whitney, calm down. These doctors are not here to put an NG tube back in."

The crashing waves of panic eased. "What's my hemoglobin?"

"You remember a few years ago when your hemoglobin was 4.8, and you were really sick?" Mom's voice was soft and soothing, but I caught the urgency. "Well, it's kind of like that now."

A normal hemoglobin range is between 12 to 15, and it's the part of the blood that carries the oxygen throughout the body and the brain. The lower the hemoglobin is, the less oxygen the brain is receiving. With the flow of the oxygen coming from the tube in my nose, my brain's ability to function was back.

I saw the hopelessness in the medical professionals' eyes. I was aware of their nervous glances. Their deafening silence gave me the real answer: This was nothing like the time when my hemoglobin dropped to 4.8—it was worse.

"Do you know your name?" the doctor asked. Had the deprivation of oxygen affected my memory of who I was?

I nodded my head, "It's Whitney."

"Where are you?" The doctor wanted to see if I was in touch with reality.

"I'm on the Hemoc floor."

"What day is it?" Was my sense of time still intact?

"It's Tuesday night."

I answered the questions correctly, but that didn't change the Mount Everest storm we were all facing—I was fighting for my life.

The ICU staff rushed me to their unit. On the way, the specialists prepared my parents for what lay ahead as the doctors had them sign releases for extreme measures. I would have to receive several units of blood, my treatment Rituxan, and an antibiotic I'd never taken, which commonly causes an allergic reaction where a person's whole body turns red. They warned my father and mother it was imperative I didn't experience any reactions to the treatments they were administering because my body could take no more trauma.

My parents were devastated to hear this news because they were painfully aware I had always had an allergic reaction during blood transfusions and to my IV treatment. Was the revelation my mom received from God of my healing preparing them for my ultimate healing—heaven?

My father and mother were directed to the waiting room, while I was taken to a room to be attached to machines. The only other person in the waiting room was a man sitting at a computer. They thought this unusual because ICU was maxed to capacity with patients. My parents were familiar with waiting rooms, so they knew there should have been more family members holding vigil for their loved ones.

Sitting, they took advantage of a nearly empty waiting room and called family and friends, asking them to pray and help me make it to the top of Mount Everest. My mother called one of her dear friends. As she shared the heartbreaking details, she sobbed. My father took the phone from her to finish explaining the dire situation.

Suddenly, the man rose from the computer and walked across the room to my mother.

"What's the child's name?"

My mother stared into the clearest and bluest eyes she had ever seen. "It's Whitney."

"Okay, I'll put her on the *Prayer Chain*." Then he turned around, walked out of the waiting room, and my parents never saw him again.

He didn't say I'll put her on my church's prayer chain, or I'll let my pastor know—he said the *Prayer Chain*. My parents never saw him in the hallway or in another patient's room, and the next day, the ICU waiting room was full.

My parents are convinced the man was an angel sent from God, because right after he left, for the first time in my life, I had not one single reaction to my treatment, transfusions, nor did my body turn red from the new antibiotic. My immune system did a complete U-turn, and I got better quicker than any of my doctors thought medically possible.

I went to the hospital on Monday, December 19, 2011. I was rushed to ICU late Tuesday night, went back to a regular room Thursday morning, and I got to come home on Saturday, December 24, 2011—the best Christmas gift ever. Two weeks later, I went back to college to finish my degree, and in May of 2012, I graduated with a bachelor's degree in creative writing.

I'd done it. My faith and the prayers from countless prayer warriors helped me conquer Mount Everest. Just as I shared in chapel, when I didn't have the strength to go to Jesus, he came to me—he literally sent an angel. I like to imagine Jesus speaking the same words to me he uttered to the woman with the issue of blood, "Daughter, thy faith hath made thee whole, go in peace" (Matthew 9:22).

And that's what I want you to grasp. A Mount Everest may form in your life, and you may face a storm while you're trying to climb, but the key is faith. You may not have the strength to come to God, but he will come to you and give you exactly what you need to make it to the top.

But there is one thought I want you to ponder. Something I learned after I experienced my mountain victory of beating a near-death experience, going back to school, and graduating with my degree. After the immediate euphoria fades and the celebrating subsides, it is normal to feel a little lost and wonder, "Which trail do I take next?"

MOUNTAIN GUIDE TO THE NEXT PEAK:

1. Have you faced a sudden storm while climbing your Mount Everest? What was it, and how did it make you feel?
2. How did you keep your faith during the storm?
3. Did you have the strength to go to God, or did he come to you? In what ways did he come to you—prayers of others? Angelic encounter?

_____

_____

_____

_____

_____

_____

_____

_____

_____

_____

_____

_____

_____

_____

_____

_____

_____

_____

_____

WHICH TRAIL TO THE TOP?

Hardships often prepare ordinary people for an extraordinary destiny. —C.S. Lewis

I sat on my front porch to watch my friend Kelli and one of the guys who served as an SLA with us drive away. Tears filled my eyes. I felt so lost. Going to school at a Christian college felt like a never-ending church camp. For the past two years, my friendships had depth and support. I had only been graduated from college two months, and I desperately missed the safe bubble it provided.

The two days my friends had come to visit breathed life into my soul. Now they were gone—I felt inexplicitly empty. No one had prepared me for how aimless I would feel leaving behind the community I had come to love and call home for three years.

Many of my friends I went to Asbury with were still living in Wilmore, the small community the university resided in or still attending the school. I desperately wanted this to be my next trail to the top of my mountain. Going back to the place I found myself would have been a dream come true. I sought employment in the area, but no doors opened, and I wasn't about to move without a plan for where my income would come from. It crushed my heart, but this was not my trail to the top.

I soon realized moving and generating a steady income wasn't simple. For someone who has a chronic illness and needs to be on Medicaid and SSI to afford astronomically priced treatments, getting a job was incredibly difficult.

When I came off my parents' insurance at the age of twenty-one, I needed any new insurance to cover my medical costs. With a weak immune system, I couldn't work and go to school simultaneously—and getting a college degree had been a priority to me. But after I graduated and sought work and tried to figure out how to launch a writing career, I soon wondered how I would be able to use my college degree. I discovered the government benefits I received were part of a system that limited its recipients more than they empowered them to succeed.

Our state's Job and Family Services and the Social Security Administration, the two government agencies that managed my Medicaid and monthly check, lacked consistency and cohesion among its staff and caseworkers. And since one agency was state and the other was federal, they did not work well together.

Everything went smoothly as long as I didn't work. But if I tried to enter the workforce and advance in life—no one seemed to know exactly how getting a job would affect my medical insurance and monthly SSI check. Much of this was because the case bank shuffled a person from one caseworker to another. I remember the first time I was offered my first adult job—as a student aide to a sweet little boy who was autistic. I met with a caseworker at Job and Family Services to see what this would do to my benefits.

"Your salary cap per month is six hundred dollars. If you go over it, your Medicaid will go on a spin down. You don't want that to happen. I wouldn't even come close to the six hundred and would try to keep your monthly income around five hundred and thirty." The woman informed me.

The salary I would make as a student aide far exceeded the six-hundred-dollar cap. I felt so grateful when the principal was impressed with my résumé and interview answers and hired me to work on Mondays and Fridays. This was the perfect solution because I calculated I could work as an aide eight days a month and remain within the parameters the caseworker cautioned me not to exceed.

Five hundred and thirty dollars in addition to a monthly SSI check would not have been a terrible amount to bring to the bank each month, but the system was flawed. I was allowed to keep the first seventy dollars of my check, and then based on how much income I made that month with my job, the government implemented a dollar-for-dollar reduction from my SSI check. I struggled to make ends meet even though I had a job. I began to see why so many people continued to stay within the system because the more they advanced, the more they were penalized.

The decision was taken out of my hands when, in the month of May, I was within eleven dollars of the amount the caseworker told me not to go over. The air immediately deflated from my lungs—the treatment I take every six months was tens of thousands of dollars. The subcutaneous treatment I took every other week was thousands of dollars. And my medications were hundreds of dollars. My medical coverage was critical. The extremely close call terrified me, and I took a break to regroup and think through what to do next because the aide job was not my trail.

A few years later, I decided to explore my options once again. I had a college degree and a purpose and calling God had given me to tap into. I reached out to a government official who passed me off to someone at the state Job and Family Services. This caseworker with the state office informed me her job was to make sure my local Job and Family Services was doing their job by sharing with constituents what program they qualified for. She would have a local caseworker call me and talk to me about a certain program I was eligible to be enrolled in.

I was finally getting somewhere—or so I thought.

I don't know why I was lulled into a false sense of security because nothing in this system had ever been that smooth. I quickly saw *somewhere* was far off when a phone call volley ensued between me and the state and local Job and Family Services, with the state caseworker and local caseworker contradicting each other. I was emotionally and mentally spent—why would I enroll in a program I wasn't sure would be administered correctly, and where I would be the one who would ultimately pay for mistakes, not the government?

I was not finding the trail to the top of my mountain, and I was beginning to feel desperately stuck. A few months after the last dead end, determination to push against the system once again engulfed my soul. I wanted MORE. I wanted fulfillment and purpose. I decided to go to Job and Family Services and have a face-to-face meeting with a caseworker and find out once and for all the income parameters I needed to remain within to keep my insurance.

"The salary caps actually changed with the type of benefits you receive. You are only allowed to make one to two hundred dollars a month."

"Seriously?" Shock filled my body. Did the government want people who needed help to feel unworthy and demoralized? If so, they had achieved their goal, because as I sat in the caseworker's office listening to her deliver low blow after low blow, worthiness and encouragement were not the feelings they were instilling in me.

"Yeah. They are really cracking down. I'd tell you not to make any more than one hundred dollars. And be careful because once you start working, you're really going to enjoy it and want to work more. I just had a client who had a chronic illness like you. She started working, enjoyed it, and started working more—making more than two hundred dollars a month—and lost her insurance. Now she doesn't know what she's going to do about her medications and treatments."

"Wow." *What a mess.*

"It's tough. But I would tell you just to not rock the boat. You don't want to lose your medical coverage. By the way, do you live with your parents, and do they help you financially?"

"Yes." Now, as a woman in my thirties, I wonder how she thought it was appropriate to ask this question. It's normal for parents to help their children who are in their twenties and my living situation was none of her business.

"Well, here's an application for food stamps. I'd really encourage you to apply and help your parents in that way. It'll lessen their financial burden."

When mom and I got in the car, the dam broke loose. "I'm so humiliated." Tears streamed down my face.

My pain caused tears to come to the corners of my mom's eyes. "Oh, honey, I'm so sorry you had to go through that. I hate that you're in this situation."

I knew some people needed food stamps to eat, and I was glad they had the option to apply for state assistance and get the help they needed to feed their families. But I believed it should be that person's choice. They shouldn't be shamed into making the decision. I went to the agency to get guidance on how to venture into the workforce, contribute to society, help the economy, and do something that made me feel like my existence mattered on this earth. Instead, no caseworker could tell me how to do that, but when it came to encouraging a recipient to become more dependent on the system, they had this skill down expertly.

No place of employment could pay me one hundred dollars a month to work, and there was no way I could take a chance of publishing any of my books and making too much in book royalties. I looked into writing conferences to get training on how the publishing world worked and to continue to learn as a writer. Still, most of the reputable writing conferences were expensive. Too much for just an SSI check that was just barely enough to cover my bills.

I felt inadequate, useless, and looked down upon. The situation I was forced into appeared to be hopeless. But what I didn't see, in the midst of the pain, was God orchestrating this season of what seemed like directionless waiting as the preparation that would lead me to opportunities and open doors for me to walk through.

One fact should be clear by now—a person doesn't just wake one morning and say, "I'm going to climb a mountain today." You must wait and prepare if you want a successful climb that ends with the summit and beautiful mountaintop victories. Researching what it takes to climb a mountain by reading books and listening to other climber's experiences, assessing whether you have the mental strength to endure the curveballs climbing a mountain can bring, getting physically fit, making sure you have the right gear for the type of mountain you're climbing, training with other mountain climbers and your guide, planning and studying the mountain and the route you have chosen to take, and acclimating to prepare for altitude sickness are just a few of the tasks you must do to prepare for the climb. Climber Greg Botzet recommends *The Climbing Bible,* which reinforces this mountain climbing foundation. Until you've prepared all you can and you're confident in your skills and ability to conquer mountains, waiting is essential—not only for safety but so you can get the most out of your experience.

That's what God was doing for me. He didn't want to have an arrow pointing at the correct trail until he knew all the right people were in place, I was prepared to climb that trail so I could receive all the gifts he had for me, and I was ready to fulfill his purpose.

My friend and *Mountain Climbers* guest, Joy Puckett, understands what waiting and right timing mean. After participating in several mission trips, Joy pursued her degree in social work with a dream. She wanted to use her profession on the mission field.

"I know people who have gone on trips, and they have traveled internationally and done some mission work and they're kind of thinking, *ok, that was it. I'm good—I'm done.* But for me, it was just still there, kind of a part of who I was," she said.

Joy wanted a different experience than the short-term mission trips, and she found it in Uganda. "I traveled to Uganda in 2016 because I wanted to see what it would be like to be there for a little bit longer term. I wanted to experience a little more relationship building to really get to know the people we were with. So I went for about four months in 2016 just to get a little bit more of a taste of what it's like to actually live for a little while in the culture and engage with the people there." Joy grinned as she recalled the joy she felt while serving others.

Joy fell in love with the culture and people, but the timing to go back didn't happen right away. After getting her master's, she moved back home to spend time with her family, but the longing and desire to go back to Uganda to serve didn't go away. So, Joy prayed and considered going back to the country.

Joy had met a counselor from an organization called Tutapona while she was in Uganda in 2016 and decided to reach out to him. "I had actually met one of the co-founders of Tutapona at a Bible study during my trip in 2016. We had consulted with him on a case we were handling with a different organization. So I sent him an email, and he said, 'Well, Tutapona takes volunteers sometimes. You should check into that and check out our application.' And it was funny because right when I got that email, I just burst into tears." Joy chuckled at the memory.

Joy processed the information for the year, trusting her heart aligned with God's will and timing. As the doors continued to open, Joy filled out the application for Tutapona. In July of 2020, I had the honor of hosting her on *Mountain Climbers* while she was still serving in

Uganda. "The funny thing about Uganda, the first time I went, was kind of a shut door moment because I had originally applied to go to Honduras for the four-month stint. And they got back with me and said the field doesn't have the capacity for someone to come right now. But our Uganda team would accept your application." Joy's head tilted to the side as she reminisced. "So, I thought, I've been to Eastern Africa before, and is it something I want to do again? In my office at work, I got on the floor and was going to pray. Probably ten seconds into the prayer, I thought, *What am I doing? Why am I struggling with this again just because the location has shifted? My desire to go hasn't shifted, and the call I feel like God has put on my life hasn't shifted.* I thought, *God, this is a trust moment. If you shut the door, then you shut the door.* So it's funny to me to look back on it—me coming to Uganda for that short time, meeting Carl, he hooking me up with Tutapona, and here we are." Joy shrugged with a smile.

Let me tell you, the waiting is tough. The preparation can sometimes be confusing. But trust me, you don't want to begin the trail until you're ready to climb it and the right people are in place, and the perfect doors have opened. What do you do in the waiting and preparation time? Pray for direction. Get in the Word. Invest in others. Serve in your church. Seize opportunities that help you strengthen and better the talents God has given you. During my waiting, I taught Sunday school at my home church, my assistant pastor asked me to write a play, I was asked to write vespers, serious plays for my home church's youth camp, and I was invited to share my story at special events. While I felt stuck, God was peppering my waiting season with special confirmations and preparation for me to climb my trail to my summit, and they reminded me of who God created me to be.

While you're questioning which trail will take you to your mountaintop victories, look out for these moments, and seize them because it's God's way of showing you how worthy you are to him. And before you know it, you'll get your "Uganda," or in my case, flannel, work boots, and a mouse.

MOUNTAIN GUIDE TO THE NEXT PEAK:

1. Have you ever felt lost or question what to do next? What emotions did you feel during this season?
2. Did you try to discover the trail that would take you to the top of your mountain but only encountered dead ends? Did it feel like more people were against you than for you?
3. How did you combat those feelings? What did you do during your season of waiting and preparation so you would be ready to climb your trail when the time came?

_____

_____

_____

_____

_____

_____

_____

_____

_____

_____

_____

_____

_____

_____

_____

_____

_____

_____

FLANNEL, WORK BOOTS, AND A MOUSE FOR THE JOURNEY?

Some journeys take us far from home. Some adventures lead us to our destiny. —C.S. Lewis

They had discovered what caused my disease. At least that's what the email said from my nurse at the NIH. My team would fill me in when I arrived for my visit, and I would meet the scientist who discovered the cause. They never went to any detail over email because they didn't want to risk their research getting scooped.

I waited with my parents in OP11, the National Institute of Allergy and Infectious Disease Clinic, my home away from home, when I was at the NIH. I was excited, but I didn't know what to expect. Was the whole reason I began my journey at the NIH happening? Had I understood the email? Did they make a scientific discovery, or did they just have a lead? If so, what was wired differently in my body? And who was this scientist working on my case, who I'd never met and didn't know existed? I was sure I knew what he looked like. He would be a seventy-year-old man with crazy white hair, big thick glasses, and look like he never left his microscope in his lab. I also secretly hoped he would have a British accent.

"Hey, Whitney, it's good to see you." My nurse greeted me in the waiting room.

"Thanks. It's good to see you too." I smiled, waiting for her to take the lead.

"Well, come on back. We have a lot of exciting things to tell you." She grinned.

"I'm so excited."

"We are too. Dr. Su isn't going to examine you right now. Your parents can come back if you want them to so they can hear everything as well."

My nurse led my parents and me to the examining room, and I noticed Dr. Su speaking to a young man in flannel, jeans, and work boots.

Who is he? Is he a patient? Maybe he's shadowing her as a high school or college student ... he looks like he could be a skateboarder.

The nurse directed us to a room, and I sat between my parents. *Thump...thump...thump.* Could my heart be heard? No matter what I heard in that tiny room, my life was about to change.

Knock, knock, knock

"Come in," I told whoever was knocking.

The door opened, and in walked Dr. Su, Helen Matthews, and the guy in flannel and work boots I saw in the hallway!

"Hello, Whitney, Mr. and Mrs. Ward. It's good to see you."

We reciprocated the greeting, and Dr. Su motioned with her head toward the mystery man.

"Whitney, I'd like you to meet Ian Lamborn. He's a student at the University of Pennsylvania, and he's getting his MD and PhD in immunology. He came to my lab to work on his dissertation, and he was given your case. And he's the scientist who discovered the gene mutation that has caused your disease. And now, I'll hand it over to him."

I could have fallen out of my chair as I worked to keep my mouth from dropping open—he was the complete opposite of what I had pictured. *He can't be that much older than me!*

Ian walked over and shook my hand. "Hello, Whitney. It's so nice to meet you and your parents. As Dr. Su said, my name is Ian Lamborn. I've read a stack of records about you about this high." He smiled and raised his hand to show the insane amount of reading he had done on my case. "So, yeah, a gene mutation is what has caused your disease. This is a novel gene mutation, we've never seen it before, and you're the first person in the world to be discovered with it." He paused, allowing us to process the intense and profound information we had just heard. "You must have a lot of questions."

With that, a game of twenty questions times twenty was played. Little by little, a bigger picture came together. Some of the news I received was exciting—my case would be the subject of Ian's dissertation. Most of it was enlightening and pieced together a lot of my medical history—I learned the gene had most likely mutated when I was in my mother's womb. Congenital disabilities such as my club feet and dislocated hips, which my pediatricians had assumed were caused by my having no room in my mother, were actually caused by the mutation. My asthma, sinus infections, bouts of pneumonia, and ear infections weren't due to my immune system taking time to build itself, but rather to the gene mutation. My short stature, the malrotation in my small intestines, and my skin issues—the gene mutation was the answer to everything. Some of the news caused an avalanche of shock and emotions to process that filled my heart and soul. At the time, I was the only known person in the world with this disease. The amazing journey I felt I was embarking on when Helen Matthews called me three years prior was coming to pass. The question was, what did this all mean?

"I'm going to get a lot of research blood from you and your parents this visit." Ian shared. "I need to see if you inherited this mutation from one of them and see if there are any hereditary connections of any kind."

"Okay. That makes sense." I told him.

"Also, I wanted to see if you would be willing to have a skin biopsy done? This is totally your decision, and if you aren't comfortable with doing this, it won't affect your care or disqualify you from Dr. Su's protocol." He assured me. "A skin biopsy is so beneficial because if we find evidence of the mutation in the piece of skin, it will tell us the mutation is in every cell of your body and therefore, dominant. Again, I want to stress, you do not have to do this." Ian said with a kind firmness.

I quickly discovered Ian had the makings of what made a doctor great—compassion and sincerity. His solemn expression and tentative voice as he explained in depth the life-altering research findings and his asking if I would consider agreeing to undergo research procedures showed me that. He told me I was not just a science project to him to help further his career as a doctor. I was a person with feelings, convictions, and reasoning. There was no ulterior motive—nothing would move forward without my consent. I appreciated this authenticity, and in turn, I sincerely wanted to do my part to help him put together the absolute best dissertation presentation possible. But it was so much more for me. Knowing I was the only known person in the world with this disease, a sense of urgency and responsibility took root in my heart.

"I want to do it," I told my team. "This will not only help me, but it'll help other patients who might be diagnosed with this disease in the future."

A couple of days later, I watched as the nurse practitioner numbed the fatty side of my bicep. "Okay, I'm going to gently place the pen against your skin. Let me know if you can feel it."

I watched, fascinated as she gently placed a tool that looked like an epi-pen on my arm. The head of the mechanism had a small, sharp, cylindrical scalpel on the end. "I can feel it just a tad."

Her eyebrows rose. "Well, I want to hear you feel nothing, so I'm giving you more lidocaine," she said in a no-nonsense manner.

The extra lidocaine did the trick, so she gently twisted the tool into my skin until she extracted a thin layer. It was amazing that this tiny specimen would have such a big impact on my life.

The hectic and stressful week ended like all my NIH visits with a wrap-up with my team. This time, Ian took the lead, while Dr. Su supervised. More and more details emerged showing the miraculous pieces of an intricate puzzle where the picture became more transparent, but there were still pieces needed to solve the mystery.

"So one really cool thing is several other labs have studied the protein associated with your gene mutation for many years. One group determined the amino acids that were critical to the protein and published a paper about it. So, by reading that paper, I was able to determine what gene had likely mutated in you. This fast-forwarded the process of determining your mutation probably by months, if not years," Ian explained.

I let yet another profound moment sink in—if my mutation had taken months or years to discover, then I wouldn't have had the *pioneer* status of being the first one in the world to be diagnosed with this novel gene mutation.

"There is actually a mouse in our lab right now, and its genetic make-up is very close to yours. We're monitoring and finding out a lot about your mutation and the possible developments it could cause as the mouse ages." Ian continued.

I chuckled. "There's a mouse in your lab that has almost my exact genetic make-up?" I clarified.

"Yeah, you should see it." One of my nurses spoke with a grin. "It's so cute and tiny. It's like a little Whitney mouse." She pinched her thumb and pointer finger together to get her point across.

Ian smiled. "Yeah, but what's astonishing is you're in much better shape than this mouse. It's weak, sickly, and its heart is not in good condition at all. You don't appear to have heart issues, and you seem to be thriving."

I couldn't contain my joy or fascination—there was a mouse in my team's lab with almost identical genes showing signs of my gene mutation being life-threatening, and yet I was the healthiest I had ever been, living life to the fullest. My heart had developed a determination, fierce loyalty, and deep protection over this research—for my team, me, and any other person who would be diagnosed with this disease. The disease and the research was bigger than me and for the greater good of many. I couldn't help but wonder if the fog was beginning to roll back to reveal the spectacular mountaintop views of my purpose?

Since we know God created the world we live in, we know mountains have existed since the beginning of time. What's fascinating is how we see mountains as majestic adventures to be conquered. A guest contributor for the *History Cooperative* wrote a piece called "Reaching for the Heavens: The History of Mountaineering." They explain that in prehistoric times, mountains were rarely climbed, and when they were, the purpose was for religious practices, such as building altars for sacrifices or studying the weather.

But, nonetheless, mountaineering was not considered a sport until centuries later. Due to his fascination with Mont Blanc, when Genevan scientist Horace Benedict de Saussure laid eyes on the majestic beauty in 1760, he offered an award to the first person who could successfully climb the mountain. This award wasn't claimed until Jacques Balmat and Michel-Gabriel Paccard climbed Mont Blank in 1786—twenty-six years later. This climb is observed as the birth of the sport of mountaineering.[1]

Once people began seeing mountains in a different light, more than twenty-five years passed before those mountains' beauty and incredible views would be explored and respected, which led to the birth of a sport that causes people to push themselves past their limits. And sometimes, we may take years to discover our purpose.

It took my *Mountain Climber* guest and sweet writing friend, Rachael Colby, years to understand and realize the unique calling God had put on her life. Rachael eloped and emigrated from Jamaica to America when she was eighteen. Being from Jamaica, Rachael is a melting pot of ethnicities. When she arrived in America, she didn't know where she fit, and because she was a woman of many ethnicities, she didn't always feel embraced by every culture in the United States. But when she married her second husband, her connection to him and his family unlocked a passion and purpose she'd always had within. "I think I've always loved seeing the underdog overcome." Rachael said with a chuckle. "I view myself as an underdog, anyway, overcoming through Jesus over time." It's through this overcoming, her calling took root.

"I've always hated injustice, and you know, coming from a country with very mixed ethnicity, there was more class prejudice when I was growing up than a color prejudice in Jamaica. But still, you know, people have looked at me and said, 'You can't be Jamaican. You're white.' I'm like no, we're a mixed people.

"In Jamaica, we have the motto 'Out of Many, One People.' And by the way, America's motto is E Pluribus Unum— 'Out of Many, One,' and we need to remember that." Rachael's solemn expression showed her conviction.

With her husband and his family having this conviction as well to fight racial discrimination, Rachael saw her purpose, as a woman with many ethnicities, to be a bridge for all ethnicities, and this is how she's chosen to use her writing ministry—for the greater good for all.

"I've been questioned by both black and white people, like, 'well, what makes you qualified to talk about race?' And I'm, like, well, I believe it's imperative that people see black and white working together—like supporting each other, not only our own cause, if you will, but supporting each other. I believe it's biblical to love one another, to help one another, to bear one another's burdens. The Bible says out of one blood make ye all nations." Rachael proclaimed passionately. "I don't really feel so much that I've chosen this as it has been chosen for me or it's chosen me. And so, here I am." Rachael grinned with contentment.

Just as it took Rachael and me many years of searching, divine appointments, and God orchestrating the details to reveal the more incredible picture of our purpose, you may experience your own season of searching, divine appointments, and collecting pieces of your puzzle God is creating for you. The season may be long. You may feel stuck, wandering, and wondering if you're moving forward. But don't quit searching for your calling, don't stop pursuing your purpose, and don't quit climbing. Because just when the aimlessness feels overwhelming, that's when God unveils your purpose. A new determination will fill your spirit, and aerial views are now within sight.

MOUNTAIN GUIDE TO THE NEXT PEAK:

1. Did you feel stuck before you found your purpose? In what ways did you feel aimless?
2. When you discovered your purpose, did you feel a responsibility to fulfill it and a sense of protection to preserve it?
3. What sacrifices did you make, and how did you give of yourself to put your purpose into action?

AN AERIAL VIEW

Definition of Perseverance (n): Continued effort to do or achieve something despite difficulties, failure, or opposition: the action of condition or an instance of persevering: STEADFASTNESS. —Merriam-Webster

I sat across from the genetic counselor at the NIH. My parents were on either side of me, a part of this appointment because the news I was about to receive would be difficult to hear.

"So, Whitney, there're several things we now know since the last time you visited, and your team wanted me to discuss them with you." She leaned forward with brows lowered. A softness entered her eyes.

I shifted in my seat. "Okay. Well, I know the last time I was here, I had a skin biopsy done. They said if the mutation was present in that biopsy, then they would know the disease is in every cell of my body." The NIH's protocol was not to discuss research results with patients through email and to share the news in person because of the traumatic impact it could have on the patient's life. I didn't know yet what my tiny piece of skin showed, and I was anxious to hear.

"That's correct. And the mutation was in your skin biopsy. I'm going to talk to you about what those results mean as well as what we now know from the blood we took from your parents." She paused for a second. "First of all, you did not inherit your gene mutation from your father or mother. That means it spontaneously mutated in you at some point while you were in your mother's womb. With the results of the skin biopsy showing the presence of the mutation, we know the gene mutation is dominant. Does this all make sense so far to you all?"

My parents and I confirmed that it did. So far, it was all straightforward. Difficult to hear, but not difficult to understand.

"Whitney, because your gene mutation is dominant, there's a 50/50 chance you will pass your disease on to any children you have. How do you feel about that? Do you think you'll want to have children knowing you could pass this gene mutation on to them?"

There it was—the piece of information she dreaded telling me the most. I could see the questions dance in her eyes—how would I react? Would this news devastate me? Would I need time to compose myself? Yes, this news had a tremendous impact on my life. It answered the mystery of why my body reacted in the dangerous and life-threatening ways it had over the years. And now, at that moment where so many questions were answered, I discovered the same solved mystery could consume by my children's bodies as well. It was clear my new genetic counselor expected any reaction to project devastation, fear, and shame. Perhaps she even thought I would proclaim I would never want to have kids—normal and understandable feelings and emotions following such a painful blow. But that's not what I felt. Fierce protection took root in my heart for my unborn children.

One of my favorite movies is *Facing the Giants*, produced by Alex and Stephen Kendrick. In this movie, the main couple, Grant and Brooke Taylor, are battling infertility. As the husband and wife discuss their desire to have children, Brooke wonders how she can miss someone she has never met.

My feelings were similar. I hadn't met my children yet, but I loved them so much I wouldn't discount their lives just because they had a disease that could give them uncertain and frightening moments. I thank God my parents hadn't done that to me because they would have taken so much away from me if they had.

"Yes, I still want to have children." My voice was strong and clear. "I have lived a good life, and if my kids have my gene mutation, they will live a good life too." I determined in my heart, right there, I would give my children their best chance at living. I would teach them to focus on the joys and cans in life, not the pain and cannots. They would have a purpose and make their mark on this world despite the limitations their disease might bring because I would instill in them the belief that they could surpass those limitations.

The genetic counselor leaned back in her seat and gave me a half-smile, which silently spoke of her respect and admiration. "Okay." She said softly.

What I didn't know was the information she shared with me was only the beginning. I was so close to my mountaintop I could see the aerial views. But the closer I inched toward the highest peak, the more I realized the most difficult and yet profound obstacles still lay ahead.

Within my story, I've shared mountain climbing applications experts have stressed are necessary to have a successful climb that leads to the top of the summit. Most of those tips have been about the physical—objects you can see and touch. The truth of the matter is you can have all the best training, purchase top-of-the-line equipment, and have the best mountain guide accompany you up the mountain. But, if you don't have one, all-important, abstract yet powerful attribute within you, you won't succeed—perseverance. Benjamin Carnahan wrote an article for *Goal. com*, explaining ways mountain climbers inspire others to reach their goals, and perseverance was on his list due to their determination to keep climbing.[1]

As noted at the beginning of the chapter, Merriam-Webster's dictionary describes perseverance as a continued and steady effort to achieve something despite difficult obstacles and circumstances.[2] Mountain climbers will experience the unexpected conditions and intense hazards the environment brings. Their strength, will, and mental capacities will be put to the test. If they don't have the perseverance to push past unforeseen limitations, they may get a glimpse of the summit without ever experiencing what the mountaintop offers.

The same is true for the mountains you face in life. You can access all the tools and recourses available to you, but if you don't allow God to perform a work in you—to plant and nurture the seed of perseverance within your heart, then when unexpected obstacles come—anxiety, marital problems, sickness, substance abuse, infertility, you'll only ever see glimpses of the summit without ever receiving the blessings God had waiting for you on the top.

Someone who immediately comes to mind when I think of perseverance is my pastor and *Mountain Climbers* guest, Dr. Calvin Ray Evans. Pastor Cal is the son of Reverend Calvin and Doris Evans, two people who were pillars of faith in the community. Pastor Cal's father founded a mission organization called Evangelistic Outreach, a ministry that helps and shares the love of Christ with people worldwide. Pastor Cal worked alongside his father after he finished college. "By '78 and '79, I was almost a field evangelist, working with the ministry, raising support for the ministry, doing what I could. Because it's hard for us to understand, people will seldom support a ministry. Sometimes people feel like supporting a man, supporting a woman. But the man or the woman may leave—ministries stay," Pastor Cal shared. Proof of that is after Pastor Cal's father went to be with the Lord, the son continued the legacy for the ministry his father started, and its impact has been eternal.

As my pastor sat in the interview giving his testimony, recounting what he and his father built in the name of the ministry and the vision that continues today, neither one of us could have imagined the obstacles he would face the next month. Almost as if the enemy was challenging his statement of ministries staying even when the man or woman behind them dies or leaves.

I watched my pastor walk to the pulpit with his Bible via livestream. He asked the congregation to turn their Bibles to Zechariah, and he opened with this statement, "Folks, I'm more convinced than I have ever been before this could well be the last sermon that I preach." He, of course, was referring to the second coming of the Lord, but his words turned out to be prophetic in another way. As he preached about the signs and seasons that would take place before Jesus came back, one side of Pastor Cal's face drooped. It became even more obvious to the flock something was wrong with our shepherd when he quickly ended the service after the altar call and rushed off the stage.

My pastor had suffered an attack of Bell's Palsy, but the congregation felt something more was going on. What we feared came true. Our pastor was sick and diagnosed with a terrible and painful neurological disease that caused numbness in multiple parts of his body. In the back of everyone's mind was whether his statement had come to pass. Week after week, we drank in the reports of how our pastor was doing. Even though we missed him and longed for his return, it was as he said in his *Mountain Climbers* interview—our church, our ministry stayed, and we were united in lifting the arms of our pastor. Our pastor encouraged us time and time again with this phrase, which he would emphasize by saying it multiple times—"Don't quit, don't quit, don't quit," and it was the congregation's turn to encourage him to keep climbing.

Even in pain and exhaustion, he did keep climbing. After countless doctors' appointments, treatments, and prayers lifted to God from people worldwide, Pastor Cal preached his first sermon at our church almost two months after the terrifying Sunday he thought could be his last. As I watched my pastor make his way to the pulpit after a season of wondering if he would ever open his Bible on that platform again, with his congregation applauding his return, I knew it was because of his perseverance he reached the promise waiting for him on the summit. The purpose and calling God had placed on his life shone through more than ever before. Several months later, during a service of restoration and healing, Pastor Cal's faith made him whole when God miraculously healed him.

My answer was to tap into the foundation of perseverance God instilled within me as well. I was so close to God's revelation of the whole picture of my purpose. While aerial views were nice and offered hope and determination, I refused to settle for those when I could have the breathtaking views the mountaintop had to offer.

Once again, I faced my NIH team at my wrap-up visit at the end of the week. After another fast-paced week full of appointments, tubes of blood drawn, and tests undergone, I was ready for my team to follow up on the difficult news I'd heard at the beginning of the week.

"The last year and a half, we've attended medical conferences and seminars presenting your case, seeing if any of the doctors present have patients who are similar to you," Ian explained. "At one of the events, I presented your case. I, of course, didn't say your name—just explained the symptoms of your disease. After the seminar was over, a man approached me and asked me, 'You wouldn't happen to be talking about Whitney Ward, would you?' It was Dr. P.," he said with a chuckle.

My mouth dropped. "Oh my goodness. He recognized me? That's crazy." I grinned and shook my head.

"Yeah, it was super impressive. And you know, we've corresponded with him for many years, so we were really excited to meet him in person."

"I'm so glad you got to meet him too."

Ian allowed a pause before he continued, "So, yeah, like I said, we've been really busy presenting your case for over a year to other doctors, hoping to find someone like you. But we haven't, and that's not normal. Usually, after the first person is found with a new disease, other patients come out of the woodwork with the disease. We know the gene mutated at some point while you were in your mother's womb, so what we can now surmise is that most babies with this gene mutation are either miscarried or stillborn."

Silence and shock.

My mom was the first to regain her composure and speak. "So what you're saying," her voice cracked with emotion. "Is that all babies are a miracle. But my baby was even more of a miracle?"

"Yes." Dr. Su said. "It's a miracle she survived the pregnancy, it's a miracle she is still alive, and it's a miracle she's doing as well as she is doing because this gene mutation is horrific. And another thing that's amazing is none of your specialists ever knew what they were dealing with, and yet, they did everything exactly right."

An onslaught of emotions hit me at once—my heart dropped at what could have been, my soul filled with a deep appreciation to God for breathing life into me, allowing me to not only live but have the profound recognition of being the first person in the world to be discovered with this disease. A sense of awe filled my heart and soul that despite the magnitude of the mountain I had faced, I had lived an abundant and full life rich with blessings.

As I sat in the big conference room, tearing up, with some of the smartest scientists and nurses I had ever met beaming from ear to ear telling me I was a miracle, I knew what my purpose was—to share my story. To proclaim that miracles are real, and God still performs them today. To encourage people with the news that if I could make it to the top of my mountains, so could they. That's what

I knew at that moment. But what I didn't know was the mountaintop views were just beginning, and they would be MORE than I could ever imagine.

And you, my friend, must grasp on to the last bit of perseverance God has planted within you as well. The Bible teaches us in Philippians 1:6 you can be confident that God will finish the good work he began in you. So don't settle for aerial views. Persevere and claim the promises waiting for you on the top of your mountain because—I can assure you—they will be MORE than you ever imagined.

MOUNTAIN GUIDE TO THE NEXT PEAK:

1. Have you ever received news that was a turning point for you—did you accept aerial views or climb past the obstacles to the top of the mountain?
2. How did you put your perseverance in action to climb past the looming obstacles? If you haven't yet, what are some ways you can persevere?
3. What promise was awaiting you at the top of your summit? What were your emotions when you discovered your purpose?

BECOMING MORE

Nay, in all these things we are MORE than conquerors through him that loved us. —Romans 8:37 [emphasis mine]

"I'm hoping to submit my thesis to defend my dissertation soon," Ian told me.

"Oh, really? That's awesome. I'd love to come," I said with a grin.

"You'd want to come to my dissertation defense?" His smile showed his surprise and disbelief.

"Yeah, totally. A lot of it might go over my head, but I'd know you're talking about me. I think it'd be such a cool opportunity." I beamed.

How many people have the chance to attend a doctoral dissertation defense where they are the subject?

"Well, I would love for you to attend. We'll try to make that happen," Ian told me.

My heart leaped with joy at the possibility. I never thought my statement would be met with seriousness or approval. When I voiced a desire to be there, it sounded far-fetched to my ears, so the last response I expected my team to have was "We want you there too, so let's try to make it happen." Over the last five years, as the only patient with this novel gene mutation, working extensively with my team, I'd developed a special bond with them. I wasn't just their patient, I was a crucial part of their team, and it made my heart soar they recognized and embraced me in this way. It confirmed the purpose God had given me. But what I didn't know was I had only uncovered a fraction of what the mountaintop had for me—there was so much MORE to come.

"Will the disease be named by the time of your defense?" I asked.

"Yeah, it will be."

"Can my name or my initials be in it?" My eyes twinkled as I joked.

Ian laughed. "That would be cool, but no. My name can't even be used even though I made the discovery. There's a scientific protocol that has to be met."

"Gotcha. Well, however the process is done, I'd love to be a part of it." Once again, I gave voice to a wild dream I never thought would be possible.

Just as I had when I expressed interest in attending Ian's dissertation defense, I surprised my team with my boldness and interest to be a part of this process. They weren't against my request but intrigued by it. The relationship we'd developed over the fact I was the only patient they could presently find with the disease, and because they knew I was a creative writer and could think outside the box for names, caused them to want this to be MORE than just a scientific find, but a beautiful and miraculous story that could bring hope to others.

"When the time comes to name the mutation, we'll see what we can do to include you," Dr. Su offered, this time with a smile.

A year passed after I had those conversations with my NIH team, and I wondered when I would ever hear from someone on my team about Ian's thesis defense or naming my disease—or even *if* I would hear from them. Just because my NIH team wanted me to participate didn't mean it could or would happen. I reminded myself the NIH operated on specific protocols, and perhaps there was some scientific etiquette that prohibited patient participation in this capacity.

The longer I waited and received no word, the more I prepared my heart for the possibility this rare opportunity might not happen. It may sound silly, but the chance to be included in the thesis defense and the naming process became profoundly important. I had sacrificed my time, energy, and strength for my NIH team. I allowed my body to experience pain and trauma to further research to help future patients and me. And guess what? I would do it all again, even if I didn't have these once-in-a-lifetime chances. I had grown tremendously as a person and a woman in the last few years, but somewhere deep in my soul, the young girl who was bruised and battered from hurtful words, shunned by others who didn't understand, and had her authenticity questioned needed to be seen and validated.

One hot day in June, my heart leaped with joy when I received an email with the subject, "Thesis Defense."

> Hi, Whitney,
>
> I hope this email finds you and your family doing well! I know you had expressed interest in possibly attending my thesis defense in Philadelphia, so I wanted to let you know that we scheduled it for Friday, September 9th, at the University of Pennsylvania. It will probably be in the afternoon. If anything changes or we get more details about the time, etc., I'll be sure to let you know. If you have any questions about the logistics of getting there and so on, I'd also be happy to help.
>
> I hope you can make it! Obviously, no pressure if you can't. Working with you has been a pleasure, and needless to say, none of this would have been possible without your help and generous giving of your time, and literally giving your blood, sweat, and tears. We can't thank you enough.
>
> Sincerely,
> Ian

When I read those words, another layer of healing took place. I felt seen and appreciated—exactly what I needed. It was okay Ian hadn't mentioned naming my disease or including me in the process. Being invited to his thesis defense was enough. But what I didn't realize was validation was on its way as well.

A couple of weeks later, once again, my heart did that free-falling jump when I read an email with the subject, "Naming your syndrome."

Hi, Whitney!

How are you? I hope all is well. We are in the midst of thinking about what to name/call your diagnosis. I know you had expressed an interest in being a part of the process, so I wanted to let you weigh in if you're still interested. I can't promise you carte blanche in picking a name (I don't even get to do that!), but I'd love to have your opinion/show you the (relatively unglamorous) procedure of naming a new disease.

A few guidelines/things to know: first, the modern/current convention for naming genetic disorders is by a descriptive acronym. The practice of naming diseases after patients (e.g., Lou Gehrig's disease, Huntington's disease, etc.) or after the discoverers (e.g., Cushing's disease, Aicardi-Goutières, etc.) is rarely seen anymore. Instead, diseases are usually given an acronym for a name, with the letters of the acronym representing key features of the disease. This serves the purpose of giving the disease a name (so it can be discussed) as well as helping doctors and nurses (and medical students!) remember how these really rare diseases present if/when they do see someone else like you elsewhere around the world.

I tend to like simpler names, but the most important thing is that the meanings of the acronym's letters are descriptive (includes important disease features), and the acronym itself is somewhat memorable (usually an existing word). If the whole process seems like mumbo jumbo to you, you can vote for some of the ones we think up!

It's kind of like Scrabble. :-) Hopefully, you get the idea. Definitely don't feel any pressure to participate. I knew you were interested the last time we spoke, and I wanted to make sure you were included as we discuss this here as a group.

Thank you (and your family) again for your consistent sacrificial support to our team here. None of this would be possible without your understanding, cooperation, time, and energy (not to mention your literal blood, sweat, and tears). We are all very grateful to work with a patient and family like yours.

Sincerely,

Ian

It definitely didn't sound like mumbo jumbo to me, nor did I view it as unglamorous. I was excited, exhilarated, and ready to play the most important Scrabble game of my life. I knew I didn't want this name to be sterile and scientific. I wanted it to have depth and meaning. I worked for hours researching, trying different combinations of words and letters that formed an acronym with the key features of my disease and that had a profound meaning, which would inspire and empower others diagnosed with this gene mutation. I submitted three names, but my absolute favorite was MAGIS Syndrome. I almost leaped with joy when I found it was an acronym that encompassed my disease's key features because I connected with it on such a deep and personal level. MAGIS means "MORE" in Latin, and I needed to hear and believe the message of this name. My gene mutation may be a big part of my life, but there was so much MORE to me than my disease.

That's the message I wanted others diagnosed with this mutation to grasp as well. But there was another reason MAGIS was so special. MAGIS referenced a Latin phrase, "For the greater glory of God." After Dr. Su looked me in the eyes and told me it was a miracle I survived my mother's pregnancy, I knew my existence and that of other people with this gene mutation were for the greater glory of God. But I resigned myself to the fact that none of the names I had submitted would be chosen, as Ian had cautioned. The honor and privilege came from being included.

wikiHow encourages mountain climbers to celebrate and be proud of the summits they've conquered, and that's exactly what we should do when we conquer one of life's mountains.[1] I have had the honor of having over forty guests on my inspirational show, *Mountain Climbers*. I have heard stories of God restoring marriage, healing infertility, cancer, loneliness, and anxiety. Men and women have overcome disease, abuse, spiritual warfare, and insecurities. Guests have shared how God showed them their purpose, how to pursue that purpose, and how they are now fulfilling that purpose. My favorite part of every episode is the joy I see on my guests' faces after telling how big their mountains were. They proclaim the mountaintop victories they are now standing upon because of the strength God gave them to climb. And the same joy I see on my guest's faces was the same joy I felt when God revealed to me the breathtaking 360-degree, panoramic view as I stood on the top of my mountain.

Have you ever watched a movie that started with the ending to build tension and fill you with anticipation and wonderment of what the main character went through to get to the victory you witnessed at the beginning? The scene gently fades to the past to show the backstory, allowing you to watch what makes this character the person they are and drives their passion and purpose. At the end of the movie, you understand what obstacles the character overcame to get to the point you see on your screen, and you can't help but celebrate with the character whether the story is fictional or true. My story is true. My mountain was and continues to be real. And now that you understand, I'll bring you full circle—back to the beginning.

September 9, 2016—I felt my heartbeat through my dress as I sat in the lecture hall at the University of Philadelphia.

This day was the pinnacle of the amazing journey I believed I would embark on when I spoke with Helen Matthews in 2010. I watched as men and women filed in, buzzing with excitement about Ian's presentation. Ian stepped to the lectern and began his thesis defense. I felt as if I harbored a thrilling secret. Sitting amid all the professors, doctoral students, and medical students, no one knew who I was or the role I played in Ian's dissertation.

I listened proudly as Ian discussed my medical journey, which included abnormal B-cells, T-cells, and how my body's messaging system didn't communicate properly. He shared about my hemolytic crises and the deformities that would be normal for any patient who had this disease. I appreciated his effort, tenacity, and his own personal mountain climb to discover my gene mutation.

At the end of Ian's dissertation, he thanked everyone who assisted him and explained he still had one particular person to thank. He revealed to the audience I was in attendance. He shared about the voluminous amount of blood drawn from my veins to conduct his research, and he spoke about the bizarre tests I endured.

"You know we choose our dissertation subjects based on how easy they and their families are to work with. We choose them because of their willingness to put themselves through tests and research. She fit both of these criteria. This woman went above and beyond and did everything I asked of her, even when she knew she wasn't obligated to do so," he said with a smile. "She totally understood that all of the tubes of blood she gave and the weird research tests she put herself through wouldn't only help her, but other people who would be diagnosed with this rare gene mutation. She is a huge part of why I am here today."

After he spoke, he bent behind the lectern and picked up a bouquet, walked over, and gave them to me along with a hug. The day could have ended there—my cup was running over with God's blessing and gifts. But Ian still had one more piece of information to present. "And we have decided to name this new disease ... MAGIS Syndrome."

I gasped and elbowed my mom and sister, "They chose my name!" I squealed in jubilant exhilaration.

I had been seen, I had been validated, and my soul rested in the contentment it felt. I had endured great pain because of my disease—physically, socially, and emotionally, but the countless victories, divine appointments, and incredible opportunities would not have come without the pain. Everything I endured was worth it, because I knew my purpose lay within the name of the being that was supposed to destroy my life. My heart bloomed with the profound revelation of what God created me to be—MORE. MORE than my disease. MORE than my pain. MORE than my mountains. If that's not worth celebrating, then I don't know what is.

I encourage you to celebrate. Celebrate your victories, divine appointments, and opportunities that lead you to the top of your mountain. I even urge you to celebrate the pain because the beauty wouldn't have followed without the pain. After you celebrate, there's one MORE important detail you must not forget to do—take in the spectacular views.

MOUNTAIN GUIDE TO THE NEXT PEAK:

1. Do you recall a time you needed to be seen and validated?
2. How were you seen and validated? How did it heal your heart, giving you that final ounce of strength to make it to the top of your mountain?
3. How did you celebrate once you finally victoriously stood on the top of your mountain?

_____

_____

_____

_____

_____

_____

_____

_____

_____

_____

_____

_____

_____

_____

_____

_____

_____

_____

MY VIEW FROM THE TOP

How beautiful upon the mountains are the feet of him
that bringeth good tidings, that publisheth peace;
that bringeth good tidings of good, that publisheth
salvation; that saith unto Zion, Thy God reigneth! —
Isaiah 52:7

My favorite song is *Mount Testimony* by the Lore Family.
I played it on repeat during a very dark season in my life.
Mount Testimony is a song about climbing until we reach the
top of our mountains. As the Lores sing in perfect harmony,
they paint a picture of the feeling and emotions a child of
God experiences as they gaze down, looking at the valleys
and cliffs that almost overtook them. They stand in awe at
the top of their Mount Testimony basking in God's gifts and
blessings, finally understanding his profound purpose in
what he has called and created them to do.

I find no irony or coincidence this song resonated
with my heart as it did, because the Lord knew the NIH
would lead me to the truth of MORE. I was MORE than
my mountains, and this powerful message would be the
foundation of my purpose and calling. My view from the top
is spectacular, and I'm in awe I'm standing here. As I give
God the glory, let me tell you about my Mount Testimony.

I've gone on six mission trips—yes, that's right, as a
woman with a primary immune deficiency, I've gone on

six. And someday, I'm going to make it seven, because I'm not too fond of the number six.

Missions have always had a soft spot in my heart, and I desperately wanted to go on a mission trip. My uncle, a veteran of many short-term mission trips, knew this and would tell me about trips he was going on where the country's disease rate was minuscule, and he thought the trip's purpose was one I could physically handle. When I proposed the possibility to my specialists, as you can imagine, they responded with "absolutely not."

However, when I was seventeen, they finally agreed to allow me to go on a trip with my aunt, uncle, and cousins to Juarez, Mexico, to meet with one of my uncle's mission partners. Juarez is close to the Texas border, and if I needed any medical attention, a children's hospital in Texas was relatively close. Because I was going with family and not a team, the schedule was light and flexible. This was a good compromise, and I treasured the chance to get a small taste of what a mission trip was. But I thirsted for MORE.

And in 2013, I got the chance. After my near-death experience in 2011, God put his healing hand on my body, and I could feel a change within. I had stamina and strength I'd never had before, and after I graduated from college, I decided to step out in faith and be a part of a mission team. My uncle was leading a group of students from Asbury and another college, Ohio Christian University (the school my cousin attended), to Trinidad. Many of my friends from Asbury would also be on this trip, and I knew this was my time, and God knew I needed this fellowship I had desperately missed after I graduated from Asbury.

A few months after I registered for my trip, paid the registration fee, and my ticket had been purchased, I had an appointment with Dr. P. He did not share my enthusiasm.

"Has your plane ticket been purchased yet?" He asked, arms crossed and expression bleak.

"Yes," I told him. "Dr. P, I don't want you ever to think I'm disrespecting your medical opinion, but there's been a change in my body. I'm the healthiest I have ever been. I would never do it if this were before 2011, but I'm different now."

He wasn't convinced, but there was nothing he could do—I was financially locked into this trip.

Not at all happy at what I was attempting, Dr. P shared what precautions he wanted me to heed while taking the biggest risk of my life. I left that appointment feeling defeated. I had always prided myself on knowing my body and having a keen instinct and understanding of what it could and couldn't handle. But after talking to Dr. P, I doubted this gift for the first time in my life, and my heart knew the real fear that I could be making a terrible mistake.

What I love about Dr. P is I have never doubted his care for me and his effort to go above and beyond to make my best interests his top priority. He was about to do this once again. My mom and grandma tagged along with me to this doctor's appointment, and on the way home, we stopped and had dinner with my cousin, who would also be going on this mission trip with me. She asked me how Dr. P took the news of me traveling overseas. I told her he was less than enthused. As the waiter brought our food, my phone rang. I saw it was Nationwide Children's and assumed my nurse practitioner was calling me.

"Hello?"

"Yes, Whitney? This is Dr. P."

My eyes widened, and I mouthed, "It's Dr. P."

Here's the significance of his phone call—in the ten years I had been his patient, he had never called me. His nurse did. Even if he didn't say it, I knew like me, he didn't like how we ended my appointment.

"Hi, Dr. P."

"I just wanted to call and let you know there's a receptionist who works here, and she has a relative who is a social worker in Trinidad. I had her call her relative to see what diseases we need to be concerned about. There's no significant risk. Just do a good job of applying the bug spray with DEET like we talked about."

"Thanks, Dr. P." I couldn't believe what I just heard.

"While I have you on the phone, let me take a look at the labs you got before you left." Silence while he looked for my results. "Okay, let's see, this is normal, oh, this one's normal ... normal, normal, normal ... Whitney, it's like your blood counts did a complete 180."

His surprise and happiness made me grin. "I know, Dr. P, that's what I was trying to tell you. I'm so much better."

"Well, I'm much more comfortable with you going now. Just stick with the precautions, and you should be fine. I'll talk to you later, and take care."

I hung up, absolutely in awe at the God-wink I just received. God knew I needed this assurance to my shaken confidence. Now I could go on this trip with peace. The eight days I was with my Asbury community again was a true gift. The way we ministered to the people of Trinidad— visiting a nursing home, an orphanage, an addiction center, a boy's prison, a school for the disabled, and putting on a Vacation Bible School for a local village—fed my soul in ways I didn't even know I needed. One of the most amazing aspects of this trip was the honor of sharing my story, proclaiming God was a God of miracles, and telling that what he did for me—he could do for them. I've traveled to Mexico, Trinidad, and Belize and had the honor of sharing my story in all three of those countries.

God has opened tremendous doors for me to share my story in the United States and to build a speaking ministry. Whether it was writing or speaking, my purpose was to tell others miracles are real, and if I can be victorious, then so can they. I've spoken at interviews, a Rotary club, women's retreats, churches, youth groups, schools, hospitals, teen retreats, chapel, and small groups. Giving glory to God and watching hope return to hopeless faces because of what God has done for me is one of the best feelings and callings ever.

The new stamina and strength that entered my body have allowed me to be active and athletic for the first time in many years. I even purchased a gym membership and began working out. My sweet grandparents, whom I'm extremely close to and have the honor to live next door to, would put out a garden each summer. Many mornings as the sun rose, I met my grandpa out in the garden to help him pick beans and corn and handle all the heavy lifting he could not physically do anymore. Never in my wildest dreams, or those of my grandparents, would I have thought I would be the grandchild who would be there to assist them like this in their golden years.

In 2016, after I had the immense privilege of choosing the name MAGIS Syndrome for my genetic mutation, God used the experience to solidify my platform, message, and ministry—I am MORE than my mountains. I began my writing journey by starting a blog called *MORE Than My Mountains*. My desire for other patients diagnosed with MAGIS Syndrome that they feel and believe the message they are MORE than their disease has happened. Presently, there are eleven known cases of MAGIS Syndrome in the world, and sadly, one little boy has already passed away from this horrific disease. This little boy was the first patient to be discovered having MAGIS Syndrome after me. Receiving the news of his passing was one of the most devastating revelations I had to process. I wondered why him and not me? It reinforced how cruel this disease could be, but I determined his death wouldn't be in vain. I would live my life to honor him. At thirty-three years old, I'm one of the oldest living persons they can find with this disease. My little MAGIS brother and sisters, as I refer to them, have embraced the truth they are MORE, and this has become the foundation of our disease.

Shortly after Ian's dissertation, I became involved in a nonprofit called the Immune Deficiency Foundation (IDF)—an organization for individuals with primary immune deficiencies to network. This opened a whole new world for me because until I became involved with this organization at twenty-eight years of age, I didn't know other people like me battling similar medical obstacles existed. Once again, I felt seen and validated, and health advocacy became another layer to my calling and purpose. Unfortunately, I had to step away from my roles with the IDF in 2019, but for a good reason. I accepted a freelance writing position with a magazine called *IG Living*—a publication whose audience is people with immune deficiencies.

Remember how I felt stuck in the broken system of Medicaid and Social Security, but wanted to explore writing conferences to learn what I could in the season of waiting, but couldn't find a writing conference I could afford?

My friends Del and Angie Duduit also began that writing journey and became involved with a new company called Serious Writer. The goal of the founders of this company is to offer high-quality writing conferences that are affordable. Del and Angie invited me to attend a conference with them in Cincinnati, Ohio. This conference changed my life—full of divine appointments, incredible writers who are now my dear friends and mentors—and set me on the course to where I am now.

A year later, another dream opportunity came my way. I was asked to be the writer for my church's youth camp vesper team. Vespers are serious and thought-provoking mini dramas performed for the campers before they go to bed each night. To be entrusted with that spiritual responsibility and to use the talents God has given me in that way was an immense honor. It's a role I fill to this day.

A few months later, I attended my second Serious Writer Conference, and I won an award for my children's picture book, *MORE Than Your Mountains*. The next year, I received an award for this book, "MORE Than My Mountains."

My views on the top of my mountain give me boldness and confidence. After being oppressed by the government and being told many times by the outdated policies it enforced within the healthcare system that I was only good enough to merely exist, I showed them I was created to do so much MORE than just exist. The government did not give me my talents, gifts, and purpose—God did. I wouldn't allow them to be suppressed any longer. Because of the treatment I received from caseworkers at Job and Family Services, I was ashamed to admit I had to receive government assistance. Slowly, I realized if I didn't speak, then change wouldn't happen. I would no longer be held at arm's length by elected officials. It was time to push back.

In 2019, I met with my county commissioner, shared my experiences, and he helped me set up appointments with two US representatives as well as a US senator while I was at the NIH for a visit. I had the honor of meeting with these men on Capitol Hill, and one of the representatives I met with invited me to sit in on a Ways and Means Committee meeting he was a part of. When a bill was introduced he didn't have to vote on, he sat with me and listened to me tell my story and concerns.

"You see, Congressman, the message people with disabilities are hearing is we're only good enough to exist. But we were created to do so much MORE than just exist." I said passionately.

"Wow, I love that. I'm going to write it down, so I can use it," he said.

That meeting was a launching pad for change. I have worked closely with the representative, his health policy advisor, and my county commissioner. These allies helped me get contacts at Social Security and Job and Family Services who are educated so that they can correctly guide me. I developed a relationship with a caseworker at Ohio's State Vocational Rehabilitation Agency, who explained to me in depth what my government benefits mean and how to make them work for me. I have the backing of elected officials, which has lifted a burden I carried for too long.

The best part is that I've been able to be a part of possible new legislation that could be presented to Congress to better the system. Because of these opened doors, I met the right people at the right time. I could finally be MORE and pursue a book contract and a literary agent without fear of losing my medical coverage. In October of 2020, I found out Elk Lake Publishing wanted to offer me a contract, and I was signed by my agent, Del Duduit, within twenty-four hours.

The Lord saw the loneliness and isolation I felt after I graduated from Asbury University and put three women in my life, Vanessa, Danielle, and Sarah, who have become my circle of encouragers and prayer warriors, filling the void of friendship I felt. And of course because of my family, friends, and church family I have, I will always be able to count on their encouragement, support, and I know they will cheer me on with every mountain I set out to conquer.

One of the most recent and beautiful callings God placed on my life was launching my inspirational show, *Mountain Climbers*. You have seen firsthand the profound impact hosting the men, women, and youth who have miraculously conquered the mountains they have faced with God's strength has had on me and others. I hope they have blessed your heart as you have read their stories throughout these pages as well.

God has blessed my ministry and allowed me to expand to have a Bible ministry, giving my guests Bibles with the inscription, "You Are MORE," for them to give to someone who needs to tap into God's strength. God furthered my ministry by allowing me to launch a Mountain Climbers merchandise line, or as I like to call it, merch with a message to get the gospel out to people who would never open a Bible or grace the doors of a church. I'm so humbled and exhilarated at what God has entrusted me to do.

As you can see, the climb was steep and treacherous, but oh, the views of Mount Testimony are so worth the climb.

I want to thank you for going on this journey with me and taking the time to read my story and what I have learned on my mountain trails. I hope my story has encouraged and empowered you, but most of all, I desire that when you close this book, your vessel will be overflowing with hope. I congratulate you on your views from the top and commend you for all the bravery and courage it took for you to make the climb—now bask in the bountiful gifts God has given you on the top of your Mount Testimony and take comfort in the fact your lifeline will be at the top waiting with opened arms.

A CALL TO CLIMB

Every mountaintop is within reach if you just keep climbing. —Barry Finlay

If you made it this far and you haven't started climbing yet, or you've stopped climbing because the mountain is too overwhelming, the time has come. This is your call to climb because this is what you were born to do.

Rest assured, you have a lifeline at the top, gently encouraging you to keep going. Trials in life may bring climbing restrictions as you ascend, but if you have the right tools and equipment in your backpack, you will climb over them to a bridge that connects you to the next phase of your climb. Lean on the team God has given you because no matter your skill or how normal your climb seems; you aren't exempt from uneven terrain and unexpected crevasses.

In fact, normalcy can instantly turn into ever-changing climbs that lead to unmarked trails, unexpected trails, or even a path to the peak you never anticipated. Take heart when you've climbed and seem to be at a crossroads—that's when your plateau of friendship comes. Allow those special people who God put in your life to be your prayer warriors, encouragers, and cheerleaders, to be your arm holders so your plateau can be a place of healing and rejuvenation. When God gives you what you need to continue to climb, make sure to shout out praise for his blessings and gifts from the mountaintop.

Be aware, though, the peaceful season of your plateau is often preparation time for you to face your Mount Everest. Many times a vicious storm is waiting for you to complicate your climb in ways you could never imagine. Don't despair, when it seems all hope is lost, that is the moment God sends angelic first aid. After the adrenaline and euphoria evaporate from conquering one difficult climb—don't be discouraged if you lack direction and wonder which trail you should take to the top. When the timing is perfect, and the right people are in place, God will point you to that purpose. This is when the atmosphere shifts and a renewed excitement fills your spirit because the aerial views tell you that you are almost to the top. While aerial views are confirmations, please don't settle for them. Keep climbing to MORE because as beautiful as the aerial views are, nothing can compare to the breathtaking views you will witness on the top.

Grasp onto the stories you've read here, look to the mountain climbing applications and techniques you've learned that can be applied to life's mountains, and take comfort in the fact this mountain didn't form without God's knowledge or approval. He knows what you're capable of when you tap into his strength. Allow the hope of God's promises and the summit views of the mountain climbers who preceded you to propel you from where you're standing, looking at the mountain to the top, looking at where you once stood, wondering how you would ever have the strength to climb. I can guarantee as you look at what you've overcome, amazement and awe will slowly warm your heart as the sunrise appears each morning, and your beginning will applaud your courage and perseverance. Raise your arms in victory and shout this truth and message for all to hear—**I am MORE than my mountains!**

ABOUT THE AUTHOR

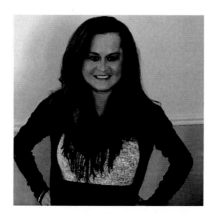

In 2013, Whitney was diagnosed with a rare gene mutation. In fact, it was so rare she was the first person to have ever been diagnosed with this illness. This disease is a primary immunodeficiency so horrific she should not have survived her mother's pregnancy. Today, Whitney is thirty-three years old, healthy, and thriving because of God's healing touch on her life. After years of research on this new disease, Whitney was invited to give the new phenomenon a name. She chose to call it MAGIS Syndrome. MAGIS is the Latin word for "more." She gave the mutation this name in hopes the meaning will give future patients who are diagnosed with MAGIS Syndrome the assurance they are MORE than their disease. MAGIS also references a Latin phrase, "To the greater glory of God." Whitney couldn't imagine a MORE perfect name because people who are living with this gene mutation are a miraculous living testament to God's greater glory. After living a childhood filled with surgeries, hospital visits, school absences, and unanswered questions, Whitney hopes that through her story, people of all ages will know despite the mountains they face, they are MORE!

You can check out *Mountain Climbers* episodes at https://youtube.com/c/MountainClimbers_WhitneyWard.

You can check out what the cute Mountain Climbers Shop has to offer at https://whitneylaneward.com/mountain-climbers-shop.

ENDNOTES

BORN TO CLIMB

1. "How to Climb a Mountain," *wikiHow,* article last modified July 5, 2021, https://www.wikihow.com/Climb-a-Mountain.

Climbing Restrictions

1. Annie Wilslowski, "Learn This: Understanding Altitude Sickness," *Climbing,* September 20, 2017, https://www.climbing.com/skills/learn-this-understanding-altitude-illness/.

2. "Hydration 101: How Altitude Affects Hydration," *HydraPak* (blog), October 17, 2019, https://hydrapak.com/blogs/beyond-adventure/high-altitude-hydration.

Not in My Backpack

1. "How to Climb a Mountain," *wikiHow,* article last modified July 5, 2021, https://www.wikihow.com/Climb-a-Mountain.

The Bridge to the Ridge

1. Tim Peck and Doug Martland, "How to Choose a Climbing Harness," *goEast,* October 22, 2018, https://goeast.ems.com/how-to-choose-a-climbing-harness/.

A NEW TEAM

1. "How to Climb a Mountain," *wikiHow,* article last modified July 5, 2021, https://www.wikihow.com/Climb-a-Mountain.

2. "The Ultimate Guide to Belaying," *Sportrock*, June 28, 2018, https://sportrock.com/the-ultimate-guide-to-belaying/.

A Different Path to the Peak

1. Jay Parks, "Climbing and Bouldering Rating Systems," *REI*, https://www.rei.com/learn/expert-advice/climbing-bouldering-rating.html.

AN UNEXPECTED TRAIL

1. "Who We Are," *National Institutes of Health*, (access late May 2, 2021), https://www.nih.gov/about-nih/who-we-are.

2. "Route Finding and Navigation for Mountaineering," *REI*, https://www.rei.com/learn/expert-advice/route-finding-and-navigation-for-mountaineering.html?series=mountaineering-skills.

THE PLATEAU OF FRIENDSHIP

1. "Organization," *National Institute of Health*, (access late May 2, 2021), https://www.nih.gov/about-nih/who-we-are/organization.

2. "How to Climb a Mountain," *wikiHow*, article last modified July 5, 2021, https://www.wikihow.com/Climb-a-Mountain.

3. "The Ultimate Guide to Belaying," *Sportrock*, June 28, 2018, https://sportrock.com/the-ultimate-guide-to-belaying/.

SHOUT IT FROM THE MOUNTAINTOP

1. Jeff Bonaldi, "14 Fast Facts about Mount Everest," *The Explorer Passage*, August 15, 2016, https://explorerspassage.com/chronicles/facts-mount-everest/.

2. Hillary Bruek, "Dead bodies litter Mount Everest because it's so dangerous and dangerous to get them down," *Business Insider*, May 29, 2019, https://www.businessinsider.com/dead-bodies-on-mount-everest-are-hard-to-get-down-2019-5.

3. Grayson Schaffer, "Five myths about Mount Everest," *Washington Post*, April 24, 2014, https://www.

washingtonpost.com/opinions/five-myths-about-mount-everest/2014/04/24/9a30ace2-caf5-11e3-a993-b6b5a03db7b4_story.html.

4. Sarah Kaplan, "After searing tragedy, Everest's deadliest route is now off-limits," *Washington Post,* February 15, 2015). https://www.washingtonpost.com/news/morning-mix/wp/2015/02/18/after-searing-tragedy-everests-deadliest-route-is-now-off-limits/.

ANGEL FIRST AID

1. History.com Editors, "Eight climbers die on Mt. Everest," *History*, November 13, 2009, updated on May 7, 2021, https://www.history.com/this-day-in-history/death-on-mount-everest.

Flannel, Work Boots, and a Mouse for the Journey

1. Guest Contribution, "Reaching for the Heavens: The History of Mountaineering," *History Cooperative,* (February 10, 2019): https://historycooperative.org/the-history-of-mountaineering/.

AN AERIAL VIEW

1. Benjamin Carnahan, "5 Ways Mountain Climbers Will Inspire You to Achieve Your Goals," *Goals.com,* April 5, 2016, https://goals.com/5-ways-mountain-climbers-will-inspire-you-to-achieve-your-goals.

2. Merriam-Webster.com Dictionary s.v. "perseverance," *Merriam-Webster*, accessed May 1, 2021, https://www.merriam-webster.com/dictionary/perseverance.

BECOMING MORE

1. "How to Climb a Mountain," *wikiHow,* article last modified July 5, 2021, https://www.wikihow.com/Climb-a-Mountain.

Made in United States
North Haven, CT
15 November 2021